Wholeness

Uncovering Self Discovery

By

John T. Meddling

Contents

About The Author

I grew up in Nashville, TN, and decided to move to Atlanta, GA, in the spring of 2002, where I am currently practicing as a licensed certified massage therapist LCMT with the specialty in neuromuscular and physical therapy. My concentration is working with traumatic brain and spinal injury patients, while serving as a health and wellness consultant. My careers vary from photography, writing, electronic repair, serving as a life coach, motivational speaking, and teaching. I am most passionate about teaching anatomy, physiology, and pathology—subjects I taught for five years at Georgia Medical Institute from 2004 to 2009 as part of the massage therapy program. I am a certified TESOL/TESL/TEFL (English teacher overseas), certified by Oxford Seminars based in Los Angeles, California. I also enjoy teaching Christian education and have taught it in one form or another for more than seventeen years. But it is my passion for health and wellness that keeps me actively involved in a variety of medical and holistic research. I am also the father of one son.

Growing up in Nashville, TN, in a household with three brothers and three sisters and both parents—always led to spirited discussions in our home. These discussions related to boyfriend & girlfriend issues, sports, and school. But the family's favorite discussions were the one's surrounding "The God Questions," which fueled our recreational time as a family. I did not always get the answers I was looking for in those talks, but these discussions sparked my curiosity to know and understand a mystical Intelligence that we called God. At the age of eleven, I knew that I would be a seeker of truth and that my search for truth would go beyond having a surface understanding. I would not be one of those people who passively accepted or believe whatever was told to me. It was seeing the diversity of beliefs within my own family that made me curious about human behavior. Because if we (my siblings) were all raised by the same parents with the same value system, why were our behavior and belief so different from one another? Why was there a difference in our perception of God?

And as a young adult, it often concerned me as to why people interacted combatively over religious beliefs, and the confusion surrounding whom or what God is. It bothered me that there was so much controversy and confusion between religions as to whose religion possessed the most accurate information about God. How is it that most religions believe in one universal God but take issue with those who differ in worship and practice? These are the type of questions that stirred my interest in human behavior as it related to belief systems—and led me on the journey to understanding human behavior and God's interaction with man.

Because of my desire to understand the unique dichotomy between human beings and an invisible God—I began surveying a variety of social and religious groups. I wanted to understand the dynamics of what forms a person's belief system—so I emersed myself into various religious communities. And it has been through the observations that I have made alone this journey of spiritual exploration—that I found a non-traditional path for my own personal spirituality. And though I've acquired a lot of knowledge in my exploration for truth—I am yet learning and evolving into a person of higher consciousness. I am assuming that my ideology about God and religion may not be considered as a mainstream belief system from religious critics—but I am hoping that writing this book **Human Wholeness- Uncovering Self Discovery,** will challenge the readers to reevaluate and reaffirm their own beliefs. I trust that this book will also motivate the readers to initiate practical and critical thinking skills.

Thanks & Dedication

I strongly believe that we are greatly influenced by those we share close company with. And if this is true—I am a compilation of some really special people that I will forever be grateful to for being an influence in my life. I have been inspired by the many of you who took time to read my weekly posts, shared your comments, and have given me positive feedback. Thanks to my students at Georgia Medical Institute, who took the time to complete the Lifestyle Surveys. Without their input, I would not have had the statistics to support many of my ideologies as it relates to relationships. Thanks to Linda George for reminding me to stay focused on my writing. Much appreciation for the McCoy family and the inspiration they brought to my writing. Linda McCoy, thank you for being my sounding board for topics and critiques. Had it not been for the supporters of my writings, I might have lost the enthusiasm to continue. Thank you for your positive influence and prayers. This book is dedicated to all of you.

Special thanks to: Dr. Reginald Turner for all your time and energy in critiquing and editing my work. Without your input and directions, I would not have adequately expressed my thoughts in a comprehensible manner. Thank you so much for helping me to deliver this ideology to the world. May

God richly bless you for the blessing you've been to me in your consistent support.

Also, special thanks to my brother Donald and **M DESIGNS** who created the original cover design. Donald, you are truly gifted, and I am so grateful and proud of your accomplishments. You have touched many lives through your artwork and ministry.

Acknowledgments

I would like to express my appreciation to the many teachers of "consciousness" and creating with the mind. Their teachings have contributed to my understanding of the active work of the human spirit and the power of thoughts. I want to express much appreciation for the online references that provided me with statistics and medical articles.

Thanks to:

Cristian C A Bodo article: The Biology of Sexual Orientation

H.O.M.E. Heterosexuals Organized for a Moral Environment.

Ann Harrington's article on the Placebo Effect

Jerry & Ester Hicks –Teachings of Abraham (The Law of Attraction) & The Vortex

Wayne Dyer –Power of Intentions

Marc David M.A. –Founder of Psychology of Eating Institute

Holly Pinafore –article: How your thoughts affect your metabolism

Mike Dooley –Thoughts Become Things (Choose Them Wisely) & Leveraging the Universe and Engaging the Magic

Rhonda Byrne –The Secret

Napoleon Hill –Think and Grow Rich

Forward

This book will touch you at the very depth of your soul. Everyone needs someone to show them how to overcome their adversity—how to reframe and rethink their challenging situations in a more positive, optimistic, and uplifting manner. **Human Wholeness-Uncovering Self Discovery** will teach you how to do all this and more.

Human Wholeness is soul talk. John Meddling's soul is talking directly and persuasively to your soul. His magnificent spirit reminds you that you have a magnificent spirit, too. He exalts you to rise up and overcome all that attempts to conquer you and instead to conquer it yourself. John teaches with tremendous wisdom how to be on top of your problems, situations, and circumstances rather than letting them be on top of you. Through this process, you learn to heal many of the broken and damaged parts of your life and restore it to a place of Wholeness.

John is a master storyteller. He writes in the gripping fashion of a best-selling novelist. He shares his own experiences of being caught in the quagmire of life's problems and tells how he swam to the edge of safety and success while never losing his humor, joy, and positive outlook on life.

He does this with a radiant, robust smile and inspires you, and teaches you to do the same.

John's lessons will make a positive, permanent difference in your life, your business, and your future. A book's value is not in how you feel when you read it but, more importantly, in how you can use it to handle your day-to-day situations, circumstances, and problems. John makes us believe that we can heal and grow. He fills us with the power of hope, happiness, encouragement, and the idea that "I am bigger than my biggest problem(s)."

This is a book that you will never forget. It will help you over and over again. I also predict that you will find the need to give it as a gift to those you love so that they, too, will be helped, inspired, and restored.

He is going to put a smile on your face, hopes in your heart, and joy in your spirit!

Reginald H. Turner, Ph.D.

Introduction

Human Wholeness- Uncovering Self Discovery is John's ideology relating to the complexity of human behavior in relationships and how the individuals' absence of self-worth immobilizes spiritual growth. He expresses his opinions as to why people struggle with the inability to make clear and concise decisions and why people struggle with their identity. He focuses on the reasons for human insecurities and how it affects the dynamics of living in higher consciousness. John expresses his thoughts on many biblical teachings that are frequently misunderstood or misinterpreted—causing those scriptures to be used out of context. His use of scriptures is made relative to these articles—and he uses interchangeable terms/names in relating to "God." Terms he uses for God are Higher Intelligence, The Essence, Creator of the Universe, Source, our God Aspect, The Subconscious Mind, Subconscious Self, and Spirit. The purpose of these various titles for signifying an intelligent source that we call God is in the hope of connecting to every reader on every level or term as they relate to "God."

His sole purpose for writing this book is to first challenge the reader's critical thinking skills and to enlighten its readers on the innate creative powers that dwell within each of us to assist in the acceleration of reaching our greatest potential. This book includes a compilation of expressions shared by individuals struggling with a variety of relationship issues and relationship dynamics—along with those who are challenged with their identity. John has interviewed, consulted, and surveyed a range of people to establish facts about lifestyles, belief systems, and cultural norms, to name a few. These individuals vary in sexual orientation, religion, social status and politics, and everyone in between. John believes that all people are seeking "wholeness" whether they are conscious of it or not. He also believes that people are as whole as they are aware and active in their responsibility to humanity. This responsibility to humanity consists of contributing to the growth and development of our society. The highest level of wholeness is reached when we commit to serving our fellow man with our talents, gifts, and resources.

Regardless of our titles, positions, age, sexual orientation, gender, or spiritual/ religious beliefs—as human beings, we all share the same basic need and host many of the same fears. We are all in pursuit of happiness, peace of mind, love, and acceptance. We all seek wholeness on different levels, and we will only discover it when we tread the waters of self-discovery.

For many years John has sought to understand his roles as a father, as a husband, and simply as a human being. He has asked, "How do I serve in each of these carnal/ human roles and yet be a spiritual individual connected to Higher Intelligence?" The complexity of being human has driven him to the exploration of self-discovery. He believes that if he grasps an understanding of his own complexity, he will better understand the people and world around him as well. So, he went on the journey of studying and interviewing people of diverse sexual orientations, ages, gender, religious beliefs, races, and cultures. His curiosity about human behavior led him to associations that heightened his social awareness.

As John engaged in diverse intercultural environments where there were differences in beliefs, he began to discover his "true self" in the person of a spiritual being. He became validated in his own belief systems and began to understand that the contrast of other people's lives was actually helping him shape his own life. So, the information that you will find in this book is a compilation of others' experiences as well as John's ideology. He simply serves as a messenger on many of the topics—but most of the expressions reflect his own ideology. Because he is ever-evolving, relearning, and breaking away from old belief systems—he reserves the right to change his opinions and views in upcoming materials. This book will hopefully cause you to engage in the process of critical thinking—something many people fail to do when understanding their own belief systems.

When we understand our individuality and live accordingly, we will eliminate some of the frustrations that we encounter in our relationships with ourselves and with others. Having a healthy perception of one's self is the foundation for true appreciation for the social world that surrounds us. Often, we find fault in the other person when our relationships fail. Unfortunately, when we fail to understand the complexity of ourselves and the dynamics of our individuality—we often misinterpret the actions of others and fail to consider their individuality. Failure to understand the dynamics of one's self often becomes the culprit for the demise for relationships and friendships.

As individuals seeking to understand one's self or individuality, we must first examine ourselves and discover what really makes us tick. We must conclude the reason(s) for our passivity or aggressiveness, dependency upon others, or independence. Why do we require so much attention, or why is it that we fail to appreciate attention when it is shown to us? What makes some people competitive and others complacent? These are just a few aspects that we might find ourselves challenged by. But this dichotomy can be implacable to any aspect of our life as it relates to behaviors that prevent us from being in harmony with ourselves and the world around us. It is in the observation of one's self that these questions should be answered—revealing the essence of our *being* that will lead us into the bliss of understanding personal wholeness. Wholeness is experienced when we understand the dynamics of ourselves first—and then share that knowledge with the world.

As human beings, we should not exist only to be led by others' beliefs, perceptions, and opinions. Humanity is beckoned to a higher level of consciousness and a greater sense of self-awareness that will ultimately deliver us into wholeness. In the articles throughout this book, John is expressing that we are indeed made in the image and nature of God, the Highest Intelligence and essence of all life. It is in the hope of this belief—that the contents of this book will enlighten and allow you to see yourselves in a more majestic, empowering, and self-loving way. Our relationships will become more productive when we obtain wholeness within ourselves. When we experience personal wholeness, we will become healed in our spirit, healed in our soul, and healed in our bodies.

Article 1

Who Am I

The question that should be asked to begin the process of self-discovery that will ultimately lead to understanding personal wholeness is "Who Am I?" Who we are from a core perspective, will vary from person to person, depending on our frame of reference and life experiences. Everything we've experienced, everyone and everything that has influenced us—has made us who we are today. It becomes a matter of being able to properly decipher these experiences in order to fairly discern and access the world around us. It is through our own lens that we view the world the way that we do. So let's begin by first establishing that as human beings, we consists of three aspects. These three aspects that underlines our human make-up are: Body, Mind, and Spirit. Our bodies reflect our physical aspect, the Mind reflects intellect, and our Spirit is the eternal, all-knowing guiding force within us.

The Body simply serves as the shell that houses both the Mind (intellect) and Spirit (the God aspect indwelling us). Our physical bodies, however, require physical substances in order to be sustained, such as food, shelter, and clothing. We, as humans, are so intricately designed that we must be conscientious of how we take care of these complex frames. Therefore, making good health decisions and **not** ignoring a healthy lifestyle as it relates to what we eat and drink with healthy activities will directly impact the quality of life we experience. For example, we know that eating unhealthy foods (foods lacking nutritional substance) can cause our thinking to be foggy. It is hard to function or concentrate on an empty stomach and expected to perform well at work or school. And as well as proper dieting, physical rest is also a crucial element to being able to function at an optimum level in a fast-paced society. And to mention that the use of any illicit substance such as drugs or alcohol can only lead to impaired judgments—is a no-brainer. And I would be remiss in addressing the danger and downfalls of living carelessly and without restraints. To be careless in any area of your life is a gamble with disaster. Though living without restraints may give you a temporary sense of freedom—I can assure you through life experiences, it is a road that only leads to mental, physical and spiritual bondage. And not just the type of bondage that lands you in jail or prison—but the kind of bondage that entraps you into a life of lack and deprivation. In my opinion, this is the worst kind of prisons for a human being to be confined by. Our life and our Body must abide by certain disciplines in order to experience true wholeness.

The Mind is comprised of intellect, logic, emotions, intentions, purpose, objectivity, desire, and opinions. It is the home of where our life experiences and frame of reference live. And too often, the decisions for our lives are made from this aspect—sometimes to our detriment when seeking spiritual answers to non-logical matters (such as matters of the heart, which is solely the job of the Spirit.) The Mind is the vehicle through which our logical decisions are made. I will dive more into this as we continue on in this article.

The Spirit is often defined as intuition, perceptivity, or instinct, and it is simply the God part of our humanity that leads humans into perfect decision-making. This aspect of our being is eternal and never ceasing. Our Spirit is the all-knowing guiding force within us that can lead us to every perfect decision if and when we learn to harness its latent powers. Our Spirit is the internal guiding force (voice of God) that navigates us into higher consciousness. It is the work of the Spirit that's beckoning from the subconscious—and awakening the conscious Mind. It is God/ Highest Intelligence communicating from within us to the conscious level of our understanding. Attempting to put it simply—It introduces the supernatural revelation to human intellect. And if we're to take away the Mind and Body by way of death., only the Spirit (or God in us) will remain because the spirit/God is the essence of who we are. I will go a step further and say that the Spirit is the God aspect indwelling our physical bodies, but is heard and understood through conscious Mind or logic. I personally believe that we, as humans, are innately more spiritual beings than we are physical beings. I believe that we existed in Spirit long before we took on physical bodies. The Bible states: *"Before I shaped you in the womb, I knew all about you. Before you saw the light of day, I had holy plans for you…"* (Jeremiah 1:5 The Message Bible). Even in Hinduism according to the Vedas, *all beings are souls* (or spirit) *and thus spiritual in nature. Though the body is temporary and eventually dies, the soul is eternal. After death, the soul is reincarnated, taking birth in another physical body or form.*

I also believe that innately we are more "God-based" than we are human-based. But the socialization from living as human beings has disconnected us from the essence of who we are. In this reality, we focus most of our attention on survival…, working, eating, clothing, maintaining shelter and etc. But our Spirit or "God aspect" has no need for food, shelter, or clothing because it is eternal, and it is our essence, and it is Source. Spirit never dies, just as God never ceases to exist. And for those who are atheists, I will express it like this: The essence (The intrinsic nature of who you are as an intangible abstract that determines your character) never experiences death even when your body ceases to exist—it continues to live on in the form of energy. In other words, the real you never stop existing; it simply transfers forms.

Therefore, to understand the relationship between our physiology, psyche, and Spirit—we should take extra care in the maintenance of our whole being. It is vital to the balance of our human complexity that we live in harmony with our whole *being* by observing the well-being of the Body, Mind, and Spirit. It is not enough to simply eat healthy to preserve the Body. In addition, taking time to relax and restoring the Mind is a crucial element in being whole as well. When the Mind is relaxed (referring to that conscious space), the voice of the Spirit which is heard through the subconscious—will then be heard in the quietness of our conscious ears.

When we bring these three components of our humanity together, analyze their relationship to one another, and gain an understanding of their dynamics, it can enlighten us about the specific areas in which we are informed. Understanding these three components of our *being* will unlock the doors to who we are.

There is also one other aspect of "Who Am I" that I would be remised to address. This hinges upon the understanding that we as human beings are a compilation of thoughts about *self*—confined in any given moment. To further elaborate, when we perceive ourselves to be in a situation—we trap that perception into that present moment, making it a reality. For example, when a person wins a million-dollar lottery—they instantly see themselves as a millionaire. But nothing has physically changed around them at that moment. That person, however, is now experiencing psychological (Mind) change in their perception of *self*. Their mindset went from lack to abundance, and the image of *self* becomes illuminated by the new reality of being a millionaire. Who we are is determined by the thoughts we hold at any given moment—and not by circumstances. We do not need a million dollars to live in the mindset of a millionaire. If we seek wealth, good health, a better job, or any other thing—we must see ourselves already possessing it. Daydream about having what you want, putting yourself in the mindset of already owning it—and it will find its way to you. **It will require you to work towards what you believe and anticipate for your life**. Your desire will lead you onto avenues of ingenious ideas that will feel like they came from outside of you—but in actuality, it is the subconscious influencing the conscious directing you towards your heart desires. So, there will be requirements of you to take actions in accomplishing your possessions. It is in the present that we are, or become, what we believe ourselves to be. *As a man thinks in his heart, so is he* (Proverbs 23:7 KJV).

It is crucial to human and to the spiritual growth that a paradigm shift about ourselves is made in each moment of our life. We must envision ourselves as possessing whatever we desire with the concept of manifesting it in the NOW! No one can determine who we are but us. The life we desire is held ransom by the beliefs we hold about ourselves. Nothing can affect us unless we give permission to it. So, live in the awareness of possessing all good things NOW! The awareness that one has of him or herself will answer the question: "Who Am I?"

Article 2

Understanding the Conscious and Subconscious *Self*

The enlightening of the conscious and subconscious *self* is the foundation of understanding where God/ Highest Intelligence becomes intertwined with humanity. People have asked me, "How do I know when God or the Highest Intelligence is speaking to me?" My answer is always prefaced with the belief that human beings are multifaceted in dimensions, but all share the same spiritual Source—meaning that we all possess the "one all-knowing spirit" that we call God. And this spirit or intelligence is wired into our *being*. It is in the awareness of the subconscious *self*—that God abides. We can identify the *inaudible* voice of God when we are able to hear the voice of concise information coming from within us—from our subconscious *self*. Sometimes this information may not make sense to our analytical minds, but we *feel* a certainty of truth about the information we receive from it. This is what the voice of God sounds like—it sounds like truth and certainty—and may not always align with our human logic.

Let us first examine four aspects of the conscious *self* which are **rationalization**, **convictions**, **perception,** and **ego**. The conscious self is the part of us that has learned behaviors as to what is appropriate and inappropriate—it consists of the values taught to us as children by parents, teachers, or anyone who influenced our life. The conscious self might be better understood as the *mind*—and this leads us to our first aspect of the conscious *self,* which involves rationalizing.

Rationalization is the action of attempting to explain or justify behavior or an attitude with logical reasons, even if these are not appropriate. And most people, as I have stated before, are prone to self-deceptive reasoning. We are naturally rational and analytical *beings* and can readily tap into this aspect because we have been taught from childhood the values that form our opinions and reasoning. And the value system that was created in our childhood becomes the next aspect of our conscious *self* which is convictions.

Convictions are any firmly held belief or opinion about any given thing or situation. What we hold or consider as appropriate or inappropriate lies within this dynamic. For example: If we were taught as children not to steal because it was bad behavior, it would be ingrained that stealing is wrong. Our conscious *self* would have adopted the belief that stealing was inappropriate behavior. The conscious self is analytical and perceives the world through the eyes of logic and makes decisions based on what it has been taught to believe as appropriateness. The logic, unfortunately, can be clouded if what's being perceived is coming from a uninform or misconstrued belief. Conscious reasoning is the natural or superficial human way of thinking. Sometimes it becomes foggy in its ability to discern right from wrong—often being governed by one's perception. This takes us to our third aspect of the conscious *self,* which is perception.

Perception is the ability to see, hear, interpret, or understand something through the human senses. There is a higher sensory that we can obtain that is beyond our *human* senses, but I will address that later in this article. But our perception is also formed by what we have been taught to believe. Of course, it is understood that everyone has their own opinions or perception about what is appropriate and inappropriate. With this being said, everyone's perception will be different from another because no two people perceive or understand things exactly the same. In addition, no two people have had the exact same experiences in life that are responsible for molding their perceptions. Therefore, our feelings and emotions become entangled in our judgments about what's right or wrong. This is where the fourth aspect of understanding our conscious *self* becomes activated through our ego.

The ego is a person's sense of self-esteem or self-importance. It is part of the mind that toggles and wrestles between the conscious and unconscious in determining reality through its own experiences. This is where debates and disagreements with others whose views are in opposition to ours are formulated. In our ego, there is little tolerance for differences, and offenses become apparent when what we have been taught as acceptable is challenged. The conscious self, because of the ego factor, can be prideful and threatened when beliefs are questioned. Feelings and emotions are weaved into this aspect of self, which subjects human beings to erroneous beliefs and misconstrued perceptions.

As I referenced a moment ago under "perception"—there is a higher sensory that's beyond our basic five senses that are found in the **subconscious self** (the place where I believe God's voice is heard). This heightened perception is an aspect that most people are yet learning to tap into. Often, we have heard the term in the religious world as "walking in the spirit" in reference to heightened consciousness. The subconscious self is a spiritual aspect of human beings. It is the chamber where God infuses us with *its* impressions—and this essence embodies all truth. Whereas the conscious self has four aspects, the subconscious self has only one—and that is "truth" or "knowing." **I am being very deliberate in restating that the** subconscious self serves as the home where God abides within humans and where God gives supernatural guidance and insight into every aspect of our lives. When God or Highest Intelligence speaks to the subconscious self—it is not analytical but simply "knowing," and it is absolute. The subconscious self when in-tuned with God (as I referenced earlier), is perfectly clear in every regard and in every situation— never requiring counseling or guidance, for it is indeed the Higher Intelligence, the God of the universe, influencing our directions. Hearing and understanding the voice of God through the ears of the subconscious self has to be learned through experiences and practice—unlike the conscious self or mind, which comes more naturally because it is connected to our life-long learned behaviors. This is why I believe people fail to hear the voice of Higher Intelligence clearly—because there is often a need to analyze from a human perspective what is spiritually being introduced. The wisdom of Higher Intelligence cannot be analyzed by the mere conscious self—for the conscious self is void of spiritual clarity in its nature. *"The natural man cannot understand the things of God for they will appear to him as foolishness—neither can he know them because they are spiritually discerned."* (1 Corinthians 2:14 paraphrased) From a Hindu expression as it relates to understanding the spiritual elements of God—*many Hindus understand God to be Brahman or the Infinite. The Infinite or God is believed to be all-powerful, and beyond comprehension because God is formless and without attributes, but manifests in form.* This is to simply say: God cannot be understood through mere human intellect or logic.

We must awaken our conscious senses to the reality of our subconscious self in order to hear the voice, the directions, and the wisdom of God. When we become more accustomed to living from the wisdom of our subconscious self—our God aspect, we will experience the peace that innately becomes us—the peace we experienced as infants. We will not find ourselves worrying over matters in this life but will live in the calmness that everything is always well with us. When we live in reality or the *knowledge* of our subconscious self, we become more at ease with the behaviors of those who oppose us. When we live in the reality of *knowing*, because we have heard and understood the voice of God within us—we are then living enlightened—and we do not concern ourselves with the opinions of those who are not enlightened. We will never have to seek out success, for it will always find us. Those who walk in the *knowing* do not chase after money, jobs, or careers because the enlightenment of *knowing* is always internally guiding you to where your success is. Living through this awareness of self is where human beings were perfectly meant to live—for we are not meant to simply guess our way through life. Life is meant to be lived by intentionality. This is how God infiltrates the consciousness of the world through a paradigm shift. We must shift from living by accident or by the whims of life—and transfer to living more intentionally. If all of humanity could only connect to the Source abiding within it, how blissful and wonderful life would be. In the next article (Article 3- **Power of the Subconscious**), there will be more specifics about how to live more intentionally.

Article 3

Power of the Subconscious

The subconscious, also referred to as the *unconscious mind,* contains all of the stored information of everything you have ever experienced. And as a side note, there are things that we have experienced or learned that may not have been taught to us but have been transferred through our DNA. To expound a little further, there may be fears, insecurities, addictions, and emotional trauma that wasn't directly our own experienced but was passed down from our parents, great-grandparents, or ancestry. Nonetheless, no matter how we come about these *unknown* experiences, they are still very much a part of us. And to push the envelope on this idea a little further, some things bottled in our subconscious may not have even come from this earthly realm but have been passed down to us from a spiritual dimension. And this is why I referenced in the first article (**Article 1 Who Am I**) that we as human beings are more spiritual in nature than we are physical. And just as ideas, opinions, beliefs, and fears can be transferred to us on a subconscious level as children—so can attributes from the spiritual realm be downloaded to us as well.

But getting back on track to understanding the power of the subconscious and veering away from being psychoanalytical., I am witnessing that most people are more focused on the material aspects of their lives rather than the spiritual aspects. We often negate the power of the spiritual forces that govern our lives that manifests from the subconscious to our conscious and into our reality. The conscious *mind* focuses on the tangible or material world of reality, while the subconscious communicates with the spiritual or unseen world. Our subconscious brings the unseen into the realm of the seen/reality. Higher Intelligence communicates divinely through the subconscious mind—for it is God or the Highest Intelligence working through us in assisting the creation of our realities. We can actually say that our subconscious is where the God of the Universe intertwines into our humanity—guiding us through the journeys of life. Therefore, we should take notice of the things we draw into our lives through our conscious or deliberate actions.

We innately possess the power to summon from our subconscious, which enables us to operate as creators in manifesting what we want. Because of our innate ability to connect with the Divine, what we think about or focus upon becomes our reality. However, we must see ourselves as divine entities operating through the human experience—understanding that we are expressions of God manifested in human form. This is why we as human beings have such a strong desire to thrive and excel, to live with purpose, to love, and to create after our kind. When we see ourselves from the divine perspective, we will empower our lives through the work of the subconscious mind and will create a life that innately reflects our divinity.

Understanding that we are innately divine (because God lives within us)—I believe that visualization is important in manifesting our realities. When the subconscious is triggered by images (whether imaginary or on a vision board)—the creation of our heart's desire is more powerfully brought into our conscious focus. The lifestyles, the love relationships, the job or careers, and the spiritual experiences that we wish to have, become more precisely manifested. The purpose of the conscious mind is to make observations, create desires, seek out strategies, and move in the direction of the things wanted. However, the subconscious is working outside of our intellect to bring into existence our desires and wishes. When we understand the concept that the unseen forces within us are in operation, aiding us in our creation, we can take pride in our deliberate manifestation of good things. But there must be an alignment of the conscious and subconscious mind in order for creation to be speedy. This alignment takes place when our consciousness (natural mind) comes into agreement with the subconscious (spiritual mind). From a religious perspective—this might be termed as *Walking in the spirit.*

When we become clearly focused, directing our attention and energy on the things we want—allowing visualization to spark that sense of anticipation—to the point that we feel we already possess the things that we desire—we will then speed up the creating process. Life is meant to be enjoyed, and we are meant to possess the desires of our hearts. But failing to understand how to manifest the abundance in our lives—will ultimately leave us unfulfilled and disappointed. We suspend our joy when our conscious mind is void of the understanding of God indwelling us. A feeling of powerlessness can taint our *sense of self* when we fail to understand the; *who, what,* and *where* of "God" from a conscious perspective. You may ask, *"Who is God?"* God is the all-knowing *Source* that lives within every living soul. *"What is God?"* God is the *Force* that drives our existence and directs our path through life. *"Where is God?"* God is found simply in the essence of our *being* or in our subconscious. This causes human beings to share in God's divinity—realizing that God lives within you. See Article 48- **Who or What is God?**

It should be noted that the manifestations in people's lives are slow or sometimes nonexistent when they fail to understand the power of walking in the awareness of their divinity. We shouldn't live in a space where we are perpetually experiencing lack and unfulfillment. We need only to live in the reality of

God's consciousness which brings all good things into our reality. After all, God lives, moves, and thinks through us—and we are empowered when we recognize it. Acts 17:28 states: *For in him* (God) *we live and move and have our being* (existence)., *even as some of the poets have said, for we are the offspring of God.*

Article 4

Reconnecting to Source

It is imperative that an understanding is established about who or what a "Source" is. When talking about reconnecting to "Source," I am speaking of connecting to God, Higher Intelligence, Creator of The Universe, or whatever name you choose that defines who or what God is to you. I do not relate to God by gender because I personally do not believe that God can be confined to gender—or to any one thing that is physical.

In order to understand our connection to Source or (God), we must maintain a comprehension of facts that, first of all, there is absolutely no way for human beings to be disconnected from the Source. God is the "Source," and is the essence of whom we all are—wrapped in human form only in experiential levels and dimensions. What I mean by *God being wrapped in human form only in experiential levels and dimensions* is best explained in this example: You own a Maserati, one of the most luxurious cars in the world—but you are unable to drive it because there is no gas in the car. Until you fill the car with gas—you will never know or experience the power and the luxuriousness of its ride. The only level of appreciation that you can have for such a fine piece of machinery is admiring it as it sits in the garage. The same is true about experiencing God, who abides within you. If you never activate the power and splendor of God within you—you're negating the wonder of God's presence. All human beings possess a quality of God, or attributes that reflect the divine nature of God—that I believe makes up the essence of our *being*. If we are unable to connect with this Source that we relate to as God—then our life will be unfulfilled—just as the Maserati that sits in a garage—can never fulfill its purpose being confined.

Now there are some who acquire more of the "perceived" characteristics of God because they have learned to master their lives through proper teaching and supernatural insight. As a result of mastering or connecting to this aspect of their *being*, they live more harmoniously, possess deeper insight, seem unbothered by life's disappointments, and possess an overall sense of well-being. Through our life experiences, we begin to get glimpses of what our God-source looks like—along with the revelation of who we are as spiritual *beings*. When we understand the relationship that we have with the God, we can then know that human beings and God are inseparable.

Since human beings are inseparable from their God-source, the question arises, *why don't we get what we need from God—and why are we found lacking?* I have already hinted towards that answer earlier, but to add—I believe that we fail to obtain the things we need or want because the communication network between us and our God-source is blocked. Since we are inseparable and are one with the Source, could it simply be that we are out of tune with ourselves? Maybe our intentions towards our creation is marred with doubt and lack of expectation? Or could it be that in failing to understand our *God's ability*, we lack the fuel to create our reality—therefore, forfeiting the things that are rightly ours—again, as in the case of the Maserati that sits in the garage that only needs gas?

Human Beings have the creative ability to draw the supernatural into the natural. Often our sense of feeling unworthy hinders the process. Many of us have been taught to believe that this sense of unworthiness is humility, but it is not. If anything, unworthiness is more connected to the lack of faith—feelings of not deserving.

If the essence of who we are is God—then how can we believe that God in us, clothed in human form, is undeserving? We must realize that when we request (by way of prayer) anything of God, we are only giving permission to ourselves to have those things we are petitioning. We do not have to ask for permission to get what we want but simply *summon* and *allow* those things to come into our lives. As co-creators with God, who lives within us—we are able to manifest the supernatural into the natural. It is God working through our humanity that brings to us all that we seek. We are not being arrogant when making these claims but walking in the awareness of "The Source" within us. Until we grasp the depths of our greatness as human beings, there will always be a lack of manifestations in our lives.

The thought of mankind being one with God may sound like blasphemy in the ears of religious people, but this ideology is referred to many times in the Bible. Jesus himself expressed this same belief in St. John 10: 30-31 by saying that "*I and my Father/God are one.*" Jesus' statement was perceived as arrogance by the Jews, so they took up stones to kill him. This is no reflection on the Jews because many people today share the same sentiment that we are not this connected to God to boast this kind of intimacy with The Creator. And if they could, some people would stone you today for making such a proclamation. The belief that humans can be one with God might sound outrageous because it has been so ingrained in us by the religious world. Religious institutions have indoctrinated the belief that we must work for God's acceptance—when in truth, we cannot ever be separated from the Source. Higher Intelligence is ingeniously hidden within our human dynamics—to the point that we are inseparable from our divinity. Until we identify with the divinity within ourselves, we will never experience the unlimited bliss and manifestation of our true selves.

Reconnecting to our Source is simply a matter of a paradigm shift of one's image of *self* and the understanding of the dynamics of the God & human relationship.

How a person perceives their life is based on the treasure they find within themselves. When we find the God within—we'll discover the wholeness of life.

Article 5

The Power of Emotions

Understanding our emotions is probably one of the most undervalued aspects of being human. When we understand the reason for having emotions, we can then begin the learning process of how to make these coalitions of feelings work for us. Let's look at some key questions about emotions that must be addressed first:

1. What is the purpose of having emotions? Emotions help us to communicate with others and the world around us, such as when we feel sad and need someone to help. Emotions also help us to act quickly when we encounter danger, as in the case of crossing a street and seeing a car coming self-protection at high speed. The sense of fear causes us to move and react quickly as a means of self-protection. So, fear serves as a means of **self-preservation**. Emotions like joy give us a sense of purpose and well-being, while more challenging emotions like disgust help us redirect what is harmful or unhealthy. Every one of our emotions serves a particular purpose. And just a side note—there are only two categories of emotions—these are emotions that make you feel good and emotions that make you feel bad. We will go into more depth with these categories later in this article.

2. How do I harness my out-of-control emotions, whether they are good or bad emotions?

A. Be aware and observant of your emotional state at all times. Always pay attention to what has caused you to feel a certain way.
B. Do not react when something emotionally jolts you. Take a moment to breathe and process how you should respond.
C. As you process your response—consider the effects, consequences, and outcome.

These three simple outlines can help you to harness out-of-control emotions, whether they are positive or negative situations. We should be aware in situations where we are considering doing something good, giving someone on the street money—should not be an act of responding out of emotions. When we are seeking the highest good for another person, we should always respond from a place of compassion but, even more importantly, from a place of wisdom and *knowledge*.

As I stated earlier, there are only two categories of emotions—these are emotions that make you feel good and emotions that make you feel bad. The names for our bad emotions are anger, frustration, anxiety, sadness, fear, guilt, loneliness, helplessness, and emptiness, just to name a few. Our good emotions are love, joy, satisfaction, contentment, amusement, happiness, serenity, joy, and fulfillment, to name the positive few. Our emotions teach us how to be social beings and how to interact and function in society. The expression of emotions one to the other is the staple to having a civilization—and this is a very powerful reality within itself. But there is another dynamic to the power that our emotion carries as it relates to our individual selves. And this is the manifestation ability that our emotions have on our lives.

Our emotions at any given time tell us where our thought process is. If only we pay attention and lend awareness to it, as I stated earlier when I talked about harnessing emotions—can we then use our emotions to manifest the good we seek in our lives? Our emotions are the guiding senses that clarify our connection to God. It is like a compass that shows us the direction we are heading in…in creating the reality we are seeking for our lives. Our emotions give insight into what we are continuously thinking about or where our "thought energy" is being focused. And when I speak of "thought energy," I am referring to our emotions following our thoughts—therefore producing our realities. When we maintain positive emotions by having a healthy outlook on life, we align ourselves with the Creator of the Universe, and this actuates the creative energies that are within us. And yes, we have the power to control, manage and maintain a good emotional state at all times. **It takes work and practice**! But these healthy emotional balances are common practices in Buddhism. The controlling of emotions prayer/meditation, exercise/stretching, and proper breathing—is one of the main teachings or practices in yogism (the teaching of yoga.)

When our emotions are in alignment with a sense "of all being well," we are more connected to God/*Source*. And in this space "of all being well" or *wholeness*—we become more sensitive and in tune with the need of humanity. It is within this space of wholeness that we realize and acknowledge that our purpose for living is much bigger than our individual desires. I know from my own personal experience that the world outside of me for a brief moment feels like an intricate part of me. This is how I believe that we create a global paradigm shift for peace and harmony. I know this might sound like a whole lot of "tree-hugging hippy stuff," but I truly believe that human beings exist to serve one another—whether we accept this ideology or not. When we serve one another retrospectively, we serve ourselves as well.

It will serve us well to understand that our emotions connect us to all humanity and, if properly managed and utilized, can direct us to supernatural guidance. This supernatural guidance cannot be mistaken or misunderstood because it is translated through our emotions. God speaks to us through the power of emotions. This is why when we witness acts of injustice in our society—we experience an array of emotions like anger, hurt, frustration, helplessness, sadness, and vengeance. Our emotions are what evoke the action for change. The Bible in Mark 11: 15-17 states: *When Jesus reached Jerusalem, He came to the temple and began to drive out those who were buying and selling there. He overturned the tables of the money changers and the benches of those who sold doves and would not allow anyone to carry merchandise through the temple courts.* We also see in the case of Dr. **Martin Luther King, who was known as a peaceful man, express anger and frustration** over the mistreatment of Black Americans. He felt racism was morally wrong and felt justified in marching for civil rights. He used his righteous indignation towards racism to effect policy change and win supporters' hearts and minds. Sometimes righteous indignation needs to take place in order to provoke change. It is God expressing through us in the form of our emotions. And these expressions are also examples of what the powerful work of emotion looks like!

All ill-feeling emotions are not necessarily bad, depending on where it is stemming from—as we can see in the examples above. But we need to be conscientious about not allowing our emotions to be carried by every little whelm. We do not sense and feel things for the mere sake of sensing and feeling—we experience these emotions because sometimes they reveal our connection to God. This is to say that sometimes it is God's source within us that pushes us towards righteous indignation. But the negative emotions that many people walk around with all day (for no good reason) are usually signaling their disconnection from the *Source*—while the positive emotions signal harmony and connectivity to *Source*. In order to have a clear channel to *Source*...negativity, hurt, anger, fear, and any other ill-emotion will have to be eliminated or managed. Unmanaged emotions will short-fuse your channel or connection from the very *Source* that sustains your well-being.

There are actually only two categories of emotions—the one that makes you feel good and the other that makes you feel bad. There is absolutely nothing in between. We are inclined to give our emotions all kinds of names, such as anger, frustration, loneliness, sadness, hopelessness, and fear. These are all emotions that we consider as bad. On the other hand, we have what we consider our good emotions, which are: joy, gratitude, hope, serenity, excitement, and love. It doesn't matter the name we give our emotions, but it is important to know that all emotions give insight as to whether we are in harmony with ourselves—and in harmony with our Source.

The power of our emotions has the ability to drastically influence our lives in whatever direction we allow it. We must make a conscious choice to be in alignment with our emotions—by maintaining that space of peace and harmony within ourselves. When we manage our emotions—we are more aligned with the nature of God, which is peace, harmony, and clarity. The wisdom of the Universe—will guide us through all of life's experiences if only we learn to manage our emotions.

Our life today is the manifestation of the emotions we managed in our past.

J. Meddling

Article 6

Courage to Face Yourself

When we, as human beings, allow ourselves to love and accept our individuality and not be judgmental of ourselves, we begin to live in the power of our *inner self*. It indeed takes courage to face who we really are. Confronting the insecurities that lie within all of us can be a challenge to our self-validation. Self-esteem can be compromised when consumed with the convictions of how we should be—judging ourselves based on others' expectations of us. Therefore, it makes no difference how affluent, impressive, or influential we appear to others when we pose ourselves to be our own worst critics.

When we become fixated on our failures, it becomes a heavy weight of unnecessary convictions. These inner convictions that we unnecessarily shoulder only lead to a sense of insecurity which pulls us out of alignment with our faith, confidence, and our *inner self*. It is within this space of the *inner self* that we connect to the Highest Intelligence— where our creativity and our power of manifestation abide. Too often, we are unaware of the insecurities we host until it's revealed—perhaps via confrontation with someone else.

Confrontation has a way of exposing our strengths and weakness—but when our weaknesses are drawn to the forefront by any given situation, we tend to try and justify our weakness or insecurity by telling ourselves that we are okay. We become self-inflicted with disillusion to "save face" (as they say) to prevent us from acknowledging our true fears and faults. The courage to face one's self is the ability to embrace and accept the fears, insecurities, and faults as part of our humanity. We are not perfect in the sense of not having vulnerabilities.

One of the dangers of not embracing and excepting our vulnerability is that we believe the lie that we are telling ourselves, that we have it all together. This is the pitfall of the ego that leads people to believe that they are invincible. And if we are in a position of authority or influence—this delusion may negatively affect all who are connected to us, including children, spouses, friends, colleagues, and subordinates, to name a few. This is especially true in a family scenario where a parent refuses to admit a wrong to a child—and the child grows up believing the wrong—to be right. And the cycle continues by producing more ego-driven, fearful and insecure people who are unable to embrace their human vulnerabilities. As parents, we should be able to say to our children that *"Even though I am the parent, I do not proclaim to be perfect."* Our children need to hear us communicate that truth from time to time. They need to know that we have fears and insecurities—but teaching them how to become triumphant in facing those fears by the example we lead. Let's not hinder the emotional and creative growth of our children by being too proud to express our inabilities. Parents must sometimes become vulnerable with their children by teaching the lessons that no one gets too old for inner growth and correction. When children are taught the value of facing the realities within themselves, they will develop a healthy social perspective about the world around them and the world within themselves. This understanding is applicable to all communities and not only in the family scenario. Because more often, we see this delusion play out with people of authority in leadership positions—where a leader becomes so inflated by their own ego or pride that they begin enforcing rules and regulations that underserve the people. This mentality reflects the egotistic need to usurp power and authority. The unfortunate reality is that the innocent and the underserved become the victims of one person's unmanaged insecurities. The fear of facing one's self is often an unconscious act of acknowledging one's own inabilities— which we all possess.

Failing to embrace and acknowledge one's own inhibitions is to deny Higher Intelligence the opportunity to manifest and express wholeness through our human form. God touches the lives of a nation or family through its leaders, but if the leaders are led astray by their own insecurities or inhibitions—so will all who follow. However, those who seek truth, transparency, and enlightenment will always find their path to inner harmony and peace. Those who acknowledge their fears, weaknesses, and insecurities will live triumphantly. We are the image in the mirror—do not be afraid to face it!

Foolish is the man who looks into a mirror and refuses to recognize the image he sees.

J. Meddling

Article 7

The Power of "Self"

I believe that the unseen realities in the spiritual realm are constantly changing and adapting to the requests and needs of human beings. The irony is that many do not recognize nor understand or give enough attention to the impression we're having on the world around us—natural or spiritual. Every day this spiritual realm which I call the *universal world* (the place where God exists within and outside of us at the same time), is expanding its arms of provision upon every new life that comes into it. God or Higher Intelligence is in constant acquaintance with the human spirit and is revealing more of itself through our human instrumentalities. When we understand that we are physical expressions of God on earth, we will be able to take our places as the conscious co-creators of the universe. The perceived mysteries of God are unfolding before our very eyes revealing who we are through the person/entity of God, as well as revealing who God is through the beings we are. We need to know that humans and God are one. The Holy Bible confirms this in St. John 17:2,1, which reads: "*that they may all be one; even as you, Father, are in Me and I in you, that they may also be in Us...*" (New American Standard). In other words, as God and Jesus are one—having the same focal point in harmony—let all human beings also possess the same mindset of harmony and "oneness." Being "one" is identified in that scripture as having the same focus or intentions. As I stated earlier—we are all co-creators with God, and all of us have the ability to bring into our reality whatever we desire. It is the God of the Universe within us, enabling us to live our lives purposefully and to manifest the supernatural realm into our natural or physical reality.

Understanding and utilizing the power that lies within the *self* will propel us to a supernatural level of living in authority. We will be able to thrive with certainty as we pursue our destiny in life. We can live as deliberate and conscious creators, knowing that the experiences in our lives have been summoned and not just encountered. Humans were not created to merely exist on the earth without having control of anything—living life by chance, or surviving on a limb and prayer. We were created to thrive and conquer our dreams and ambitions—to live life in abundance with joy and bliss. Unfortunately, many will not gravitate to this higher God-given call because many will never get beyond the survival mentality. The *inner self* must be elevated to God's consciousness or God-mindedness, which is the ability to think creatively as God. When we esteem our *inner selves*, we, in turn, exalt the God who resides within us. The Holy Bible references this fact: "*You are from God's little children and have overcome them; because greater is God who is in you than he who is in the world.*" (1 John 4:4 New American Standard.) We are not diluting the authenticity or

55

power of God by esteeming ourselves. But rather giving credence to our connection to divinity.

When we fail to understand the power of *self*—we tend to accept whatever comes into our reality. Some might think that it is humility to simply accept unwanted things into their lives—but this way of thinking is degrading to the intelligence and *mercy* of God, who enables us to create the reality that we desire for ourselves. It is God that commanded the first *perceived* humans, Adam and Eve, to take dominion over every living thing that moved on the earth (Genesis 1: 28)—and this included taking charge over themselves, their conditions, and their realities. Our duty is to take the gift of life and multiply it in the unique way that we see fit as individuals. In the Bible, Mathew 25: 14-30, Jesus tells the parable of the three servants or managers who were given different talents (or amounts of money to invest) for their master while he was away on a long trip. And just like one of the characters in that story, many of us are wasting the "talent" of our life by not managing or creating abundance in our own lives. Please understand that when I am speaking of abundance, I'm not necessarily referring to getting rich and having a fleet of cars or living in mansions. I am simply referring to manifesting a life that represents more of what you want out of life. It may not be materialistic things that you are seeking, but it could be better relationships with friends or family or finding a significant other.

Having a life that better represents you may include being able to travel or build or expand a business. It really doesn't matter what your creation is—as long as it's a creation that gives you fulfillment and purpose.

But there are so many people who feel that someone else would do a better job managing/creating their lives for them. This lack of understanding of the creative power of *self* is why people seek out other to give them directions for their own lives. We often give the responsibility of making our lives better to others, like a pastor/clergyman, a parent, or even a best friend. We give more credence and value to them for knowing what is best for us. But the truth of the matter is that no one is better equipped with what's best for you but you. No one can know as specific as you what best creates a harmonious and fulfilled life but you. Consequently, when we place the authority of our lives into the hands of others—we are often directed onto a path that is not in harmony with our true desires. When we are afraid of taking control of our own lives for fear of failing or making a mess of it because of a wrong decision—and therefore render it to another, then we forfeit our divine creativity.

We are born into this existence as creative *beings* that have been equipped with our very own navigation system for this life. But some of us become homogenized from our true divine nature with the fears projected upon us by others who may be unsure of their own creative ability. Many have forgotten that their responsibility in this existence is to experiment and enjoy all of the splendors and experiences that come with learning who they are as co-creators. I do not believe that the Creative God of the Universe is holding us hostage to a man-made belief system, critiquing our every move and action. Nor do I believe God to be an angry entity who's keeping an account of the bad and good that humans do. However, I do believe that every human soul is given the power to orchestrate their own destiny through self-perception. We are created and infiltrated with the wisdom that comes from the highest of all intelligence—that intelligence being God. So, let's take joy in basking in the fullness of all that our lives have to offer us—and let us enjoy the developing gifts that reside within all of us and through all humanity.

If we are to imitate the greatness of Higher Intelligence, we must first identify with the power residing within ourselves—and live in the reality of that power.

J. Meddling

Article 8

Improving Your Life by Organizing Your Surroundings

In a class discussion about self-improvement, a student asked me, "Mr. Meddling, what has been the most important factor for improving your life?" Without reservation, I answered, "Organizing my surrounding." Most people will never see the relevance of an organized environment as it relates to an improved life, but as we organize our personal living space, we also systematize things in our psyche. In my observation, people who live in cluttered surroundings usually have problems with managing their finances, managing their time, making clear and precise decisions, and being disciplined with eating. This lack of organization can be a prelude to the mindset of the people who fail to complete or even start tasks in their life. Disorganization is definitely a mindset or mentality that hinders many people's ability for creativity. When we are mentally cluttered with unfinished projects or weighed with emotions such as anger, fear, bitterness, and anything else that affects us emotionally—it can and will hinder our drive for progression. Most would not consider emotional weights like anger, fear, or bitterness as hindrances related to clutter—but emotional clutter, in my humble opinion, is the worst of all. When our physical and emotional space is disorganized, they often weigh as *incompletes* in our psyche. These *incompletes* can hinder our ability to be creative and move forward. Incomplete tasks are marked in our subconscious as failures, leaving us with a sense of not being able to achieve them. This is the reason why many lack the confidence to start anything new because the *old* or *unfinished* tasks lie before them unaccomplished. Holding a grudge, for example, is a form of an unaccomplished task because, in the emotion, something has not yet been settled. To further collaborate the effects of anger alone, Emotional decision-making can impede not just the outcome of a decision but the speed at which you make it. Anger can lead to impatience and rash decision-making.

The *essence* of who we are seeks harmony and well-being—and there is a loss of well-being when our negative emotions guide our decisions. Not only is our decision-making cluttered, but it has also been scientifically proven that people who harbor unforgiveness, hatred, prejudice, and any other vice that causes ill feelings—tend to have poorer health than those who do not.

Individuals who lack organizational skills typically have problems with maintaining a healthy diet—so it's no wonder that poor health is associated with ill feelings and unhealthy dieting. It takes a certain level of mental discipline to eat properly. Poor dieting leads to poor energy levels, which leads to poor exercising habits, which leads to poor health, which leads to a potentially shorter life. Of course, I'm not saying that every unorganized person is in poor health, but I do believe that our surroundings affect our ability to be mentally clear and mentally disciplined. I believe that the discipline we as individuals wish to achieve in our lives should first be reflected in our personal surroundings. I believe that our ability to be successful in life is directly connected to the harmony of our environment.

Not only can diet be affected by disorganization, but relationships are also affected by cluttered-minded individuals. This is not to be taken as an insult but simply means that the person whose surroundings are unharmonious is often out of balance with their *inner self*. It is through the *inner self* or soul that communication and directions for our lives transcend from The Universe/ God, who gives us our wholeness. When people are out of harmony with themselves, in some regards, they're often out of harmony with the world and people around them. This usually relates to hoarding emotional clutter. Once again, this is not to say that ALL unorganized people are out of touch with the world around them or that they all have unharmonious relationships, but to simply point out that disorganization lends to many other areas of disconnect and non-accomplishments.

Harmonizing our environment to our creative s*pirit* brings perfect synergy to the body/mind connection. This transformation can ultimately unclutter and connect us to our divinity. We are always affected on a spiritual level by our surroundings (people, places & things) because the things around us feed into our human energies. Therefore, we should strive to maintain that inner peace by organizing our surroundings. Organization perpetuates the inner peace that opens our awareness to the creative Intelligence of the Universe. The creative Intelligence within us organizes the material world around us. This creative Intelligence is God manifested in the *inner you*. Therefore, the world and the environment that surrounds you is your creative work.

Article 9

When Manifestation Is Slow

It can be exhausting and even frustrating having to wait on something that you feel you must have right now. It is especially exhausting and frustrating when you have poured your time, energy, and your heart into believing and expecting something or someone to come into your life—yet nothing manifests.

When we are deeply anticipating something, and it doesn't come alone when we expected it—we can become quickly discouraged. Questions of our worthiness or the pureness of our faith are challenged, so we lose heart, thinking that we've done something wrong to cause the Universe not to respond to our request. We often hear people say as a means of reservation that *if it is God's will* or *in God's time*, things will happen for us. In this instance, we settle for the reservation to pacify, not getting what we want on command. But the statement that *if it is God's will* or *in God's time* is usually a despairing resignation to not putting in the work of maintaining faith and/or expectation. And yes, there is work in believing, having faith, and maintaining expectations. But often, people feel that they are not yet deserving of what they are petitioning the Universe for. There is often the false belief that we have to earn our way *or right* to receive our manifestation. The mindset of having to be good enough to receive still haunts *religious* thinkers. We are not on this earth to prove our righteousness but to live out our human experience with joy and accountability. And yes, we should be accountable to the laws of the land and respect the human dignity of one another. Respecting and having honor towards our fellowman does not take away from our own enjoyment and bliss in life.

But when we lend ourselves to the false belief that we are not good or righteous enough as being the reason for lack of manifestation—we negate the power of faith and belief. Please understand, that we as human beings are not trying to win brownie points with God—for we do not exist in this world to prove our worthiness or to reach a higher level of righteousness. We are "righteous" in this very moment because we are born innately righteous. And I know what the *religious thinkers* might be saying; *Behold, I was brought forth in iniquity, and in sin did my mother conceive me.* (Psalms 51:5 ESV). This scripture is specifically speaking of King David, whom scholars say in reference to this text that if the Jewish history is true (and we have no reason to believe otherwise), David's own father and family believed that David was born as a result of adultery. This is why David himself writes, "*I was brought forth in iniquity, and in sin, my mother conceived me.*" So, we must understand that the context of this scripture relates solely to King David and should not be generalized. And for those who are

Christians, consider 2 Corinthians 5:21 *He made Christ who knew no sin to be sin on our behalf so that in Him* (Christ) *we would become the righteousness of God* [**that is, we would be made acceptable to God and placed in a right relationship with Him by his gracious, loving kindness].** Amplified Bible (AMP) **NOTE**: I am using Biblical references because the majority of my audience is Christians. But for Hindus, *salvation comes in realizing that everything is one, and that everything is in union with Brahman* (God) *and is one soul with the universal soul.* This is to say, that the Hindus believe (as I also believe) that there is no need to strive for acceptance from God, because you are already a part of God—and God a part of you.

Now that I have gotten the religious references out of the way…, Therefore, in our present state as human beings with faults, failures, and imperfections—we are still the expression of God in human form that exist in this earthly realm to live out the human experience as expressions of God on earth. I believe our true purpose is to live our natural lives with the supernatural assistance of the Universe already abiding within us. We are to simply live our individual lives in harmony with God, who resides harmoniously within our human frames. This is to say that we should live in harmony with our inner selves.

So, when manifestation is slow, there are usually only a few factors involved. The first is what I relate to as conflicting beliefs. A conflicting belief is when your personal belief system is in conflict with what you want. For example, if you desire to be a millionaire but you believe (maybe on a subconscious level) rich people often become rich by cheating and defrauding, but you are opposed to unscrupulous dealings in order to be successful—that would be a conflicting belief for you. Your framework of thinking would have to change to *"Rich people work hard and honestly to achieve their success, and I am willing to work hard and honestly to gain my success."* And with this mindset, you are now in congruency or agreement with your personal belief system, and you are ready to manifest the things you desire. So, your desires cannot be in conflict with what you believe in your heart. The beliefs that dominate your emotions are the ones that will govern your manifestation. Your belief system dictates the emotions associated with your faith which will consequently affect the manifestation. We will not manifest productively if our belief system is in opposition to our inner convictions. Our beliefs and the emotion associated with those beliefs must be congruent with one another. When these premises of belief and emotions are in conflict, we often get a mixture of what we want and what we **do not want**— but never manifesting exactly what's desired.

The second factor is not focusing clearly on the desired manifestation. Too often, we are distracted by our current circumstances that dictate our emotional *frequency,* which affects the creative process. Our focus or imagination helps us to bring a clear view of what it is that we truly want. This is where I believe vision boards and daydreaming play a role in the creation process. Having a visual of what's desired heightens the belief and expectancy of the thing wanted. Having this visual also gives us a sense of ownership even when we do not yet possess the object of desire. This is a very basic understanding of automotive sales. The salesman allows you to drive the car, work the controls, and in some cases, allow you to keep the car overnight to get a sense of ownership of it. The salesman usually asks the potential buyer, "Can you see yourself in this car?" Once we commit to liking that car and seeing ourselves in it, the salesman closes in on the sale. The Universe does the exact same thing. When the Universe sees that we have a strong, focused interest in something, the Universe/ God goes to work to bring it to fruition.

The third component of slow manifestation, but not necessarily the last factor, is the lack of desire. There are many reasons that people lack the desire to have anything better. Some may feel a sense of unworthiness, while others are unwilling to exert the energy needed to obtain their prize because it requires too much work. Others might feel that life is not meant to be abundant, so in that lack of understanding, they settle for whatever comes into their life. Yet, many others may simply lack patience and become discouraged in the waiting process. Lacking desire will destroy the need to daydream or to have the imagination of a life that is grand. A lack of desire can and will destroy one's need to have a vision for their life. This is why so many people simply exist in life but never truly live life. Their life is aimless, meaning that they have no goal to reach or vision to fulfill—and "*Where there is no vision, the people perish*:" (Proverbs 29:18 KJV). Where there is no vision, people will cast off the restraints of the law—and the law I speak of is the universal law that all mankind is made in the image or *spirit* of God. We are ALL innately divine—possessing the ability to be great and to do great things. But if there's no desire, there will be no creative energy that will ultimately lead to a life of true fulfillment. The absence of desire—is where we perish in our complacency. However, we are able to heighten our desire by simply focusing or even pretending by means of daydreaming about what we want. Heightening desire can help us regain the clear focus needed to manifest the things we are seeking. Heighten desire provides the magnetic attracting power that brings the unseen realities into the tangible realm. It gives us the motivation to seek diligently. Not standing still simply waiting for something to fall into our laps—but to actuate the work that's needed to bring about the manifestation.

Desire is the component that sets the pace of human life. This is to say that (in most cases that I've observed) those who have much are those who have desired much. On the other hand, those who experienced lack and deprivation in their lives lack the tenacity to strive and work hard for what they want. Some even lacked the desire to possess more than what they have because they believe that humility would be lost if they achieved success.

There is a direct collation between desiring to work hard for what you want and obtaining. This does not mean that all work is physical in its pursuit of obtaining, but it can also be a spiritual work stemming from the supernatural realm. For example, the exercise of thinking outside of the box, thinking in God consciousness, or in the awareness that you, like God—have the ability to create your own world. Being aware and understanding that God is residing in you— is a spiritual work within itself. The Universe will never let you down if only you send the clear message of your heart's desire. Never give up on your goals or dreams because the Universe is always creating the world around you—but through you. The world, even as you perceive it to be.

Article 10

Overcoming Abuses

Often when we think of overcoming abuses, we think of someone who is the victim of some sort of drug addiction, violence, or someone who has mistreatment imposed upon them. Of course, these are all abuses, but I have found that some of the worse cases of abuse are self-imposed. In this article I will be addressing both self-abuse and the abuses that are imposed upon another. I will begin by talking about self-abuse as a result of not understanding who you are.

I believe that people are often more critical and more torturous to themselves than anyone else could ever be. When we as human beings fail to identify with the fact that we are powerful and creative beings, with the assistance of the Higher Intelligence—we commit self-abuse. Because failing to recognize the authority we possess as spiritual, creative beings causes us to subject ourselves to bad habits and addictions that are not of our intentional creation. None of us would purposely place ourselves in a compromising situation that would in-bondage our creativity. But what's unfortunate is that many of us do not understand how we attract and self-impose these abusive situations into our lives. Adults who are—and remain in abusive situations are often victims of themselves long before they become abused by someone else.

Abusive behavior of one's self stems from the lack of understanding one's true essence. This oversite is what I believe to be one of the most profound reasons that people battle with insecurity—and leaves them blinded to their true purpose in life. When we fail to understand our true purpose, self-abuse is almost inevitable. What I mean is that a person may spend ten or more years of their life in and out of toxic situations like relationships or settling for jobs that do not showcase their strengths. I am referring to those individuals who *settle* into these situations—and are too frozen by fear to orchestrate a change. Sadly, these individuals are imposing their own abuse. They have not figured out how to get off that ole merry-go-round of *I can't do any better*. They also lack the awareness of their own divinity through the Higher Intelligence.

On the other hand, those who abuse others are also unaware of the divine authority and power that they possess within themselves. Abusers feel the need to physically impose their power upon another in identifying their own authority. The one who abuses others is just like the one who abuses themselves in that neither understands that they are victims unto themselves—being governed by their own fears and insecurities. And their healthy perception of *self* is lost in that same fear and insecurity. Therefore, the act of controlling another is a manifestation of fear. The abuser (whether self-imposed or imposing upon another), does not realize his/her lack of connection with the elevated and spiritual aspect of their own *being*. But if there was recognition of one's true essence—the aspect of our divinity, there would be no need or desire to control another. Recognition of one's divinity is what I believe to be the greatest paradigm shift in humanity.

The abused person, on the other hand, is also the recipient of their own inner fears. This is especially true if they remain in the abusive situation. When the abused person is elevated to a higher consciousness of *self*, they will love themselves enough to change their situation. And sadly, their love for themselves may not be their motivating factor for orchestrating change—it might be someone else's dependency on them that forces the change in their life. One example (in a critical situation) is the dependency of a child upon its parent for protection. In this case, the abused person is forced to make strategic changes—not for the sake of self-preservation or self-love—but for the love and protection of another—being their child. That parent or person, will not live in the deception that things will automatically get better. When a person become aware of their true worth and value (which is an acknowledgement of the *God aspect* abiding within), they will always make the right decision.

Problems do not automatically improve or become corrected in abusive situations when no proactive decision is made. Usually, the fear element of what the abuser might do if they (the abused person) become

72

proactive is often the crippling factor that fuses them into the situation. The abuser and the abused are both victims living out the manifestation of their own inner fears. One is thinking about or dreading being abused, while the other is thinking about or dreading not being respected as having authority. Both are creating the manifestation of abuse because of the attention given to what's being dreaded. One is dreading being abused, and the other is dreading not being respected or in control. Neither may be thinking in terms of the word *abuse*, but nonetheless, creating that reality.

Thankfully, we as human beings are given the unique ability to survive the most threatening of situations—and this area of abuse is no different.

Overcoming abuse, whether the *abused* or the *abuser*, a person must come to the knowledge of who they are as a spiritual, creative being, and this will, in turn, lend confidence and power to the *inner self*. When the *inner self* is validated, firmly standing in the awareness of being a co-creator with Higher Intelligence—there will be no need to control anyone or to be controlled. We are all comprised of the intricate aspects of God—the highest intelligence. When we understand that the nature of God resides in us, there will be no need to feel subordinate to one another, for we are all creative beings.

Those who abuse the world around them have already first devastated the world within themselves.

J. Meddling

Article 11

Codependences

Years ago, when I served as a counselor—I encountered individuals who were challenged with moving forward after experiencing a relationship break-up. I empathized with how hard it was for people to move on after being committed to a relationship for so many years. Many of the women I counseled during that time found themselves attempting to hold onto men who no longer wanted to be with them. I even encountered several men who were having a real challenge accepting the fact that they were losing their women. I noticed both men and women alike were trying desperately to hang onto relationships that could no longer stay afloat. I observed that many of these individuals often felt the need to remain connected to the other person in some way or another—either by friendship or some other means of association. I suspected they were hoping that the other person would reconsider and offer a second chance. Nonetheless, I would ask the question—"why do you feel the need to stay connected to them when they no longer want to be with you?" The answers were usually something like this: *Even though we are no longer a couple—because we have so much history and they really understand me, I need their friendship.* I observed that this reference to staying connected because of years of shared history had become the mainstream reason in many of these cases. I also realized that many people would stay in unhealthy relationships because of the familiarity they had with the other person—regardless of how toxic the relationship might have been. And all the more when children were involved.

Emotions are connected to all relationships, no matter the dynamics of the relationship. Nevertheless, if one is to become or remain whole as a person—they must emotionally release a person when they are no longer wanted.

Codependency in a relationship, by definition is when the relationship becomes more important to you than you are to yourself. It is a sign of codependency when you are trying to make a relationship work with someone who has no interest in it. This is a one-sided relationship. And to further elaborate, codependency is when a person who is codependent finds no satisfaction or happiness in life outside of doing for the other person. They stay in relationships even when the other person intentionally does hurtful things to push them away. A codependent person will often do anything to please or satisfy another—no matter the sacrifice or degradation. Sometimes these one-sided relationships can end in tragedy, as we often hear about in the news. Fortunately, most codependent relationships do not end in tragedy, but they do hinder people from living the full and rewarding lives they could be enjoying. Codependency becomes a serious issue when a person is unable to function in a healthy emotional and spiritual manner. We are social beings needing community, but we should not depend upon the existence of another in order to function in a healthy and whole manner.

Codependency exists when one fails to understand the innate endowment given to them by God. This is a dynamic that is only understood in one's exploration of *self*. We should always be on the journey of learning that we are spiritual beings endowed with greatness. This understanding of *self* gives us the confidence that our individual lives are more than the relationships that we're in. Living in the awareness of whom we are as spiritual beings empowered with the greatness of God gives us insight into the potential that lies within us. We cannot allow ourselves to fall victim to the pseudo-belief that our lives lie in the hands of another. Instead, we take control of our relationships (or failed relationships) by moving forward with our lives. By moving forward, we are then reconnecting to our ambitions and goals—which often get sacrificed when in a relationship. This is why it is commonly termed "*losing yourself in a relationship*."

There are many signs of codependency that are often overlooked as simply being a part of people's behavior or personalities. Some signs of codependency are:

- When a person stays in a relationship with someone who is self-absorbed or uninterested in the relationship to the point where only one initiates getting together or showing interest toward the other.
- When a person needs someone to make a decision for them about their own life or affairs.
- When one consistently needs another to validate their worth and value as a person.
- When a person frequently requires someone to push or encourage them into doing things they know they should be doing.
- When one person plays the out-of-control person so that they get the upper hand in possessing control over the other as a means of getting respect.
- When a person depends on others to tell them what's right or wrong or what's best for their life.
- When a person is afraid to take on new ventures alone.

There are others' behaviors that could be added, but they will all stem from one basic need—the need to have someone else do for you what you can do for yourself. And I am assuming that we differentiate children or handicapped dependent individuals are not a part of this equation. They would be considered codependent because of their dynamic of being a child/minor or physically or mentally unable to do for themselves. This is a different case altogether.

But for the rest of us—the Universe has supplied each of us with everything that we need for our life journey. It is wired into our spiritual DNA and intertwined into our humanity. We are our own masterpieces waiting to be chiseled out of our own experiences. The life we desire is held ransom by the beliefs we hold about ourselves. We are our own devastation or our own master creation—the volume of our worth lies within the perception of our ability. We need only to look into the mirror of the *true self* and reiterate the greatness endowed upon us by God. We are the manifestation of God in earthly form, designed for greatness, endowed with divine wisdom, empowered by love, and infiltrated with independence. Our need for validation is simply to fan the flames of our ambitions. And the validation that we're given from others—only makes brighter the light that is already within us. And the desires that we already possess for our own lives—are only made stronger by those who lend their support and acceptance.

Article 12

Why Should I Be Selfish

Being selfish is often looked upon as a negative thing, but as we define its meaning, the term can be appreciated and not be looked upon derogatively. To be selfish is to have a sense of one's self—to be connected with one's sense of need and desires or to look inward at one's devotion to self. Being selfish is an expression of self-love or self-consideration. In our awareness of self, we determine and make decisions for what we believe to be best for us. The sense of one's own need is the intricate part of our internal mechanisms that provide us with the ability to survive and exist. This awareness of self is like a built-in compass—guiding and directing us in life decisions. It can also be understood as our garment of protection— for, without a *sense of self*, our insecurities and weaknesses are exposed to those who may not have our best interests at heart. Unfortunately, there are "takers" who thrive on those who are emotionally infirmed or passive. We have all probably used the expressions *I have to watch out for me* or *I'm taking care of number one,* and *I am only responsible for my own self.* All of these statements reflect a healthy awareness of self— for this is how we survive as individuals.

Often those who lack a healthy sense of self-love or self-consideration are thought of as passive, weak, or having low self-esteem. On the other hand, there are those who are generous, benevolent, and always seeking to assist others (even if it is in tales denying their own needs) who border on the characteristics of being codependent. These individuals give in order to be accepted because…, being accepted validates their worth. They often value themselves by taking the subordinate role in all of their relationships. Their need to please everyone else and placing their own needs on the back burner is for fear of "falling out of others' good graces." This is usually an unconscious act on their part. I believe when a person continuously denounces their worth by putting others before themselves—it begins to fester a sense of disharmony within. In this case, people often become resentful towards the ones they give too much of themselves to. And on a conscious level, they may not even be aware of the self-deprivation that they're exhibiting through these actions. Hidden or unconscious hostility towards others can cause a person to unconsciously turn on themselves inwardly. I have observed people acting-out destructive behavior because of their guilt or self-anger—for allowing others to take advantage of their good nature.   And some of these self-destructive behaviors have manifested into overeating, bulimia, promiscuity, drug abuse, alcoholism, and other disorders. And it may not even be understood by the individual why such behavior has begun to govern their lives. This self-deprivation is exhibited when a person gives more of themselves to another than what is comfortable. Teen age girls who try to impress or fit-in with their piers often fall into this category. Or young adults facing college trying to take on a major that they have no personal interest in—only to please their parents, also fall victim to this dichotomy.

Relative to a relationship—the individual that gives more of themselves than what's comfortable—may also give more attention and consideration to their partner than to themselves. When people continue to neglect their own needs—whether those needs are material or emotional—it often causes the *"giver"* to feel frustration or contempt. When the giving of one's time, energy, or love goes unreciprocated, the sense of *self-love* diminishes. Please understand that this takes place on a very gradual scale, so I may sound a little extreme to some—but I am looking at the accumulative process.

So, we must live in awareness and understand that being selfish is simply our sense of self-preservation which grants us clarity of our innermost needs and desires. We can form healthy relationships in a social environment as well as our internal personal environment because we understand who we are and what we need to feel whole. For this reason, we should not settle for what we do not want in a relationship—or in any other aspect of our lives that we have the power to change. There are more than enough people in the world who are in harmony with our own desires without having to settle. Settling is only the resignation of the fulfillment of our needs and desires. Not being selfish and denying ourselves dilutes and extinguishes the wholeness of whom we are meant to be. We only encounter frustration and anxiety in not being ourselves or the person we want to be at any particular moment. It is through our awareness of self that we acquire the objectives of our lives—breeding the confidence to trust in our own decisions and not living by the opinions and expectations of others.

Being selfish actually helps us with developing self-confidence. And self-confidence helps us in choosing the best mate for ourselves. When we are clear-minded about who we are and what we desire— we will be clear-minded about what we need from our potential mate. We will choose someone who will meet our needs and who shares our core values. I believe that we only attract those who are in the same vibrational realm we are in. I also believe that we are what we attract, and it is through the consideration of one's self or the act of being selfish that we order our lives by allowing ourselves to be devoted to our own wishes and desires.

The act of being selfish can be a fulfilling experience when we maturely understand this concept and the empowerment that it lends to the practitioner of it. Just as the world and the cosmos have balance, so does this concept of being selfish. We will discuss this balance in Article 13, entitled **The Gift of Consideration**.

Article 13

The Gift of Consideration

Giving attention to one's self and being devoted to your own personal need is a healthy way to live, as I discussed in the Article 12 **Why Should I Be Selfish**. But there is a synergistic mechanism to this ideology. And what I mean by "synergistic mechanism" is that even though I am an advocate of being selfish, as defined in the previous article—I also believe that there is a balance to every action and behavior. One can not be too much on one side of the fence in order to live harmoniously. We must take into account that when we are a part, of any kind of a relationship—be it romantic, platonic, business, or friendship…, our personal needs are often found in the giving of consideration to another's desires and wishes. For example: As an employer, I was asked by my employees for an increase in hourly wages. I considered how much it would cost me as a small business owner to give these raises. Granted, my employees were deserving of what they were asking, so it wasn't unreasonable. Still, I wasn't initially *feeling* favorable toward making that decision—but when I rethought the situation and considered how much I needed these skilled employees and how deserving they were of a raise, I had a change of heart. My objective and desire for my thriving business were to maintain a smooth-running organization with happy employees who knew how much I appreciated them. And if giving my employees a raise to heighten the morale so that they would be more dedicated to their work—then it would be worth the *consideration*. So, in meeting their needs I ultimately got exactly what I wanted for myself and my business—while appeasing my employees at the same time. This action is what I term "The Gift of Consideration." Giving consideration is the same as compromise. And when we compromise, we can often get what we want by meeting someone else's needs. When we aid in helping someone reach their goals (no matter how small of a goal), we fortify our own sense of fulfillment. That act of consideration creates a connection between us and the one we're assisting—often creating a deeper sense of loyalty between the two.

Though I firmly stand on the belief of self-consideration and self-devotion as I mentioned in Article 12, **Why Should I Be Selfish**, I also ascribe that self-love is validated when we are able to invoke the consideration of others. I believe that one aspect of our personal happiness is birth from a spirit of generosity—and those who give to others are expressing (on a subconscious level) a sense of abundance in their own lives. However, this is applicable to those who give "freely" from their hearts—not feeling pressured or obligated. I've observed that some of the most unfulfilled people in the world are those who hoard everything to themselves. As human beings, we are designed to be helpers to one to another and not to merely thrive alone—if we are to experience true wholeness. Our ability to consider one another's needs causes us to be co-creators in universal harmony. Isn't this how ants create their large colonies in such a short time. If you kick over an ant-pile today—by tomorrow they would have re-built it. This is because of the productivity that comes with having unity.

As co-creators of our world, we must stay connected to our cause for all of humanity in order to fulfill our purpose here on earth. What is our purpose here on earth...you might be asking? I personally believe that our purpose as human beings are to elevate ourselves (to and on whatever level that looks like) while assisting others in their elevation. I strongly believe that we have a moral, civil and spiritual responsibility to one another as human beings. We must be able to identify and *seek* to meet the need of the people in our lives. This does not mean that we are obligated to give to everyone that asks of us, but we should live with a *sense* of consideration—being willing to help as seem reasonable to us. This consideration involves more than giving on a tangible level but also on an emotional and spiritual plane as well.

The Gift of Consideration should be freely given as any gift is, and not for the purpose of reciprocity or manipulation. People often find themselves discouraged when they give to someone who's close to them—only to discover that reciprocity isn't given. We should never give out more than we are willing to freely give. Only give what you can afford to give away—and again, I am not speaking only materialistically but in every aspect of your giving. For example, do not expect someone to love you the way you love them—do not expect a person to spend as much money on you as you spend on them, and don't expect a friend to empathize with you, as you spend empathizing with them. The point is that none of us give to the same degree because our value systems for how to give will differ. Do not frustrate yourselves by expecting someone to be like you because none of us give of ourselves the same. Nor should we give from a sense of obligation or necessity because this type of giving does not come from the heart. It will only leave us feeling remorseful, angry, or frustrated. When we feel trapped into giving out of a sense of obligation, it lends to a feeling of "being used" or "taken for granted." When we feel "used" or "taken advantage of," we lose that deep sense of wholeness. But when we properly give (giving from a place of feeling that we have more than what we need)—we increase our joy, fortify our peace and restore our love for *self*. We feel best about ourselves when we give out of a spirit of abundance and gratitude. The Gift of Consideration should always feel good.

When I think of the good, I desire for myself—but give it as an offering to another, it becomes the most powerful gift of all—it becomes the Gift of Consideration.

J. Meddling

Article 14

Finding Your Answers Within

Since the beginning of civilization humans have been on a mission to understanding the meaning of their lives. Our quest for understanding our purpose has been on the forefront of our journeys since antiquity. But because of the modern times we live in—we seek answers from a plethora of platforms that gives us 'oodles and oodles" of information that derive from other people's opinions. And these are opinions coming from individuals who are just as perplexed about their purpose, and the direction for their lives, as we are.

While many forums of information can be found through the internet, in self-help books, and in group discussions on self-awareness—many fail to search within themselves for the directions concerning their own lives. There is absolutely nothing wrong with seeking direction through these various means of information. When you are a seeker of truth—you will find yourself on a vast road of exploration. But we should never lose sight of the internal wisdom found within ourselves. In fact, the answers that you receive through the advice of others should only lend confirmation to what you already sense deep down within.

I would dare say that most of the "deep" answers that we seek for our lives are spiritual in nature. This is to say that—usually what we seek in reference to direction for our lives—is not particularly found in the natural or material realm. The essence of our *being* (what makes us who we really are) cannot be fulfilled or satisfied with material things such as cars, homes, jobs/ careers, or even a relationship. The things that are most essential to life are found deep within our *inner self*—our subconscious intelligence, which holds all knowledge. This intelligence that possesses all knowledge is what I term as the *God aspect* in operation within us. This God aspect or God force within us has the answers to our relationship's issues, our personal growth, our prosperity, and any other questions regarding our humanity. This wisdom lies within every human being. Unfortunately, we give more credence to the opinions of others who typically are trying to solve our problems with natural or tangible solutions. And as well-meaning as they might be—these solutions that they render doesn't even work for them. And many of these same individuals who are trying to be helpful—lives are in greater shambles than our own. They may not even believe or have confidence in the advice they're giving to you.

We make prayers to God as if God is somewhere out in space—and not observing the truth of God dwelling within our own *being*. We look for the answers from other human beings rather than listening to the still, small voice within our own hearts—the voice of our own subconscious—the voice of God. We often seek supernatural wisdom but find ourselves embracing carnal knowledge. We long for truth but often settle for a lie. And we do not purposely get ourselves into this "fix" or intentionally get bad advice from bad sources. It becomes an act of convenience, meaning that we accept whatever advice that requires the least amount of energy in order to obtain.

However, I do believe that God uses human instrumentalities (others people) to give us direction and instructions in certain situations. This is why we have specialists like doctors, lawyers, plumbers, electricians, auto mechanics and etc. But when relating to matters of our personal growth and direction—our total reliance should never reside on someone else…, because we are spiritual beings connected individually to the wisdom of God. We should weigh the instructions of others against our own hearts. The direction that is meant for someone else may not be the direction that the "*God in you*" is leading you in. The advice that they give you might be good advice and may work perfectly for them, because that is the *God in them* speaking to them. The God of the universe does not have only one voice. What I mean is that God could lead two people with the same exact problem in two separate directions—which goes back to my previous point that the Universe can whisper different solutions for every individual. But if you are considering implementing the advice and wisdom that others share with you, remember that their advice and wisdom should always agree or be in harmony with your own spirit or with the God force that directs your life. As a conscious creative being, only you know what's best for you. The Bible even states a truth about us having divine knowledge and wisdom. In 1st John 2:27, it reads: *"But the anointing which you have received of Him abides in you, and you have no need for anyone to teach you…* (New American Standard). Once we understand the *"Him"* in this verse as being God's knowledge abiding within us—only then can we appreciate the fact that all we need already resides within us. Therefore, when we learn to trust our own intuitions, we are learning to trust the God within us. Paracelsus who was a German- Swiss scientist said it like this: *"For God who is in heaven, is in man. Where else can heaven be, if not in man? As we need it, it must be within us. Therefore, it knows our prayer even before we have uttered it, for it is closer to our hearts than to our words."* And if I can paraphrase Paracelsus—he was simply saying that whatever we need—the answer is already within us before we ever ask (end quote). And as we practice relying on that *knowing* within us—we're training our *conscious mind* to hear the subconscious (the voice of God) on a regular basis.

What many might consider as the unadulterated *truth*, actually resides within all of us. But the problem is that we do not trust our own intuition (the voice of God) within us. It really doesn't matter what name we give God or whether we believe God to be male or female, spirit or energy—the wisdom of God resides in all of us. But those who live in consciousness (aware of God within them) live a more purpose-filled life than those who do not. Most people believe in a God or a Higher Power but have not learned how to connect with that Power that abides within them. This Intelligence is constantly supplying us with all the wisdom and knowledge that we need to experience the joy of life. For us as human beings, it's simply a matter of clearing the communication lines to hear clearly the instructions for our lives. Our lack of confidence in ourselves, and in our decisions—disables the Intelligence of the universe from communicating clearly to us. We must believe in ourselves and in the power that resides in our human frames. So, faith is a major component in allowing us to tap into the Source that's within us.

People also fail to get the answers they need because of the mentality of unworthiness they live in. If we believe ourselves to be unworthy of having the wisdom of the Universe within us—we will always be dependent on someone else to provide us with spiritual guidance. We will find ourselves relying on preachers, fortune tellers, mediums and whoever else we believe to have divine knowledge, to guide us. Most people are generally taught that God responds to our faith, but if we are trusting to hear from God outside of ourselves, then we are not projecting the faith and confidence we proclaim to have. We must have confidence or "faith" that God is capable of speaking directly to our own hearts. And when God does use someone to give us instructions—it should be an acknowledgment of what we're already feeling and thinking. A *truth* presented by anyone should only confirm what is already known or sensed in the heart of the one who seeks that truth. Everyone will not be given the same exact *truth*. What's true for one person may not be the truth for another—because our experiences with life vary on multiple levels. Therefore, God provides answers to us in a way that we can relate—sometimes using our personal experiences in life to sort out *our truth*.

The answers we seek for the direction of our lives abide within us and not in another. Let us learn to love ourselves and the *God's presence* within us—creating the atmosphere to hear clearly the inaudible voice of the Intelligence of the universe. God is ever guiding us in life—but let us become quiet in our soul—hearkening to the still, quiet voice speaking in our hearts. Let's find our answers—by finding God within ourselves.

Article 15

Dealing with Jealousy & Loss

Jealousy is a common emotion that often raises its head in relationships. There are various areas in which people struggle with jealousy, and many people are not even aware that jealousy is the root cause for many of their relationship struggles. When we feel jealous, it is a false sense that there is not enough for us, or that someone or something can be taken from us. In a relationship, it's a sense of not getting what you feel belong to you—i.e., love and affection, respect and honesty, time and attention, or anything else one might deem important to a relationship. But jealousy is not confined only to relationships. In this article, we will also explore the general aspects that jealousy can affect.

Believing that the universe lacks the sufficiency to supply everyone's needs, including our own, is a terrible misconception. The universe is always extending the unimaginable overflow of "good" into our lives. But, no matter how much the universe extends this overflow, there are many who are unaware of its provision. We must understand that Gods' universal provision is extended to us all—but many fail to recognize it because they do not value themselves as worthy of God's provision. They fail to see their own value as an individual, and they fail to see the value they hold in the eyes of a universal God. They do not understand that the universe is actually living, breathing, and abiding within them. The universe (or God's) purpose is to supply our individual needs—and has therefore internally wired each and every human being with the ability to live a life that is fulfilling—a life of wholeness. All that we need currently exists within us—for we are complete and lack nothing. Our lives would be fulfilled if we could only grasp the reality that we are co-creators with God, who abides within us—helping us create our own destinies.

All of that may sound good—and it's good to know that God has my back—but how does that help me deal with feeling jealous or dealing with someone who leaves me? How do I get over not feeling slighted when my significant other deprives me of affection, attention, or love? That's the real question, right? Well as I stated in the beginning, that feeling jealous is a natural emotion, but we must determine that we will not be dictated by our emotions. Jealousy, like any other emotion, is simply our subconscious rising to the conscious level, making us aware of our focal thoughts through our feelings. It is the undergirding of our emotions that we're lacking something that's wanted. But we can become self-fulfilled and not be dependent upon another to fulfill us. Yes, it is a great undertaking to get to the level where things like jealousy, anger, frustration, bitterness, and all other ill-feelings, have no control over us. But it is possible for us to live outside of the dictates of our emotions. If only we can rise to the level of awareness and gravitate to the concept that our thoughts become our realities, we will understand that absolutely nothing can be taken away from, or denied us. Understand that nobody or nothing enters or leaves our lives without our subconscious permission. And what I mean by this is that before we ever physically enter into this world or physical realm as a human being—we have been prepared to deal with every encounter in life. And I know this may sound a little far out there. But consider how a tree stems from something seemingly as minute as a seed—but within that tiny seed is a tree that will withstand raging storms and high winds for ages to come. The tree that was once a tiny seed has everything within itself to survive all that it must encounter—and we, as human beings, have the same tenacity as that tiny seed. We are brought into this world with the highest level of survival skills—survival in every regard is innate to us. We are divinely given the ability to create the reality we desire—even when others withhold what we feel should be rightly ours—i.e., love, affection, and attention. As humans, we have a built-in "bounce-back" mechanism wired into our DNA. We can handle and survive, literally anything. And taking control of our emotions are no different.

Because we are the creators of our own lives, no one can prevent us from creating the reality of feeling loved, appreciated, and respected. But let me be real for a moment—because I hear what some of you readers are thinking. What if my mate, friend, acquaintance, boss, or family member give what's rightly mines, to someone else—don't I have a right to feel jealous? And the answer is YES! You have a right to feel jealous, angry, hurt, betrayed, wronged, and any other emotion that you choose or encounter. No one can tell us how to feel in any given situation. But the point I am making is that you "consciously" choose to shift that emotional disposition by re-wiring your thoughts about what you're feeling. This doesn't mean that you ignore or do not address the issues with the person who is depriving you of what is rightly yours. You by all means should get this issue off your chest and talk about it. But after addressing it—and while waiting to see the change or adjustment in behavior (whatever the case may be)—consciously move your thoughts in a more harmonious direction. A direction of thought that allows you to feel at peace, with a sense of wholeness—is where you aim to be.

If we experience a "break-up" in a relationship—we may feel jealous because we're losing someone *whom we feel* rightly belonged to us—but we must understand that just as we have the right to make choices to leave or stay in relationships—so do others. Often a break-up is a sign that it is time to move on and explore new avenues of happiness. Try not to take it personally because the other person is also on a journey in their life to find happiness. We all have the right to explore the world—and the other people in it. This would be the perfect time to ask one's self the questions—*why am I feeling jealous, and what do I perceive is being taken from me*? When you make this evaluation, incorporate the *knowing* that nothing meant for you can be taken from you except with your permission. You may be thinking that "*I am not giving this person permission to walk out of my life—we have children together!*" I am not saying that giving *permission* is "telling" someone it's "Okay" for them to walk out of your life. What I am conveying is that giving permission is simply *releasing* a person if they choose to leave—no matter how much it causes you hurt. The reality is that we cannot force or *will* anyone to stay with us who wants to go. We do not have the power or the right— because if we did, it would be a direct violation of their own free will. And the Universe will never violate someone else's *will* to satisfy our desire.

Let the chips fall where they may—knowing that God truly *got your* back. This is the mindset you must adopt—this is the mindset of progressive thinking. This way of thinking will empower you to move on. There's no need for anger or revenge in these matters—even though anger might surface. If anger or any other ill emotion arises, do not try and suppress the emotion with the intention of trying not to feel it. Sometimes we must allow ourselves to feel the hurt and pain—in order to get to a better emotional state of being. It takes grieving the loss of someone who has walked out of your life in order to move forward. So, embrace whatever emotion you feel at that time—but, do not dwell there. Our emotions should never be suppressed—we should allow ourselves to feel what we feel. This is a process of grieving that is natural. However, our actions should be tempered with harmony.

We must remember that in relationships, others have a right to change their minds—and their decision might be that you will no longer be a part of their life. You might be left feeling abandoned or betrayed. Unfortunately, you will have to deal with the disappointment of releasing that individual from your life. We should also understand that we have no control over anyone's life but our own. When we live in the awareness that all we encounter in life is only an experience that is added to the wholeness of our *being* in this earthly realm—that it will become an easier transition through difficult situations like these.

The harboring of jealousy (and any other ill emotion) will only hinder the flow of joy in our lives. Incorrectly dealing with our ill emotions will taint our ability to trust again in others. We should not allow ourselves to hurt needlessly when relationships do not work out the way we want them to. We must anticipate the changes of life. When an unwanted change, such as a break-up takes place in our lives, we must understand that the *change* does not define who we are as individuals. Often, we feel defeated when people walk out of our lives—or when we lose houses, cars, jobs & careers. But if we release people and things and not focus on these situations as a loss—but merely a transition, we will experience human wholeness. This is the wholeness that comforts and gives us peace when all seem to be lost. The Bible speaks of this kind of comfort and peace in Philippians 4:7— "*and the peace of God, which surpasses all understanding, will guard your hearts and your minds in Christ Jesus.*" (New American Standard Bible). You do not have to be Christian or even religious to benefit from this verse. The principle is simple: The Universe always finds a way to bring joy and comfort back into your life after every storm.

Jealously is a fear of loss—but the awareness that the Universe supplies all of our needs is the antidote. The one who focuses on abundance and well-being— manifests the same into their reality.

J. Meddling

Article 16

Telling Your Body What You Want

We have heard the motto of the United Negro College Fund that says, "*A mind is a terrible thing to waste.*" There is a deep level of profoundness to this statement because it is through our mind/ intellect—that governs the activities of our reality. The mind houses the human perception, consciousness, and logic in order to make sense of the world around it. It also has the ability to shift us from the natural to the supernatural—from the tangible to the spiritual. But not wanting to sound so clinical—the mind can aid us in good physical health. And seeing that we are co-creators with God in creating our own realities—we have the ability to change our physical condition through the power of perception. We can make a demand on our bodies to be healthy and whole. There are other factors to this creative power that we all possess—that I will discuss a little later.

Telling your body how to function is not a new concept, theory or ideology. Ann Harrington's article on the Placebo effect suggests that patients heal faster when they surround themselves with positive reinforcements. This is also why placebos work for so many people—when a person believes that the "sugar pill" is real medicine for their particular illness, they become better simply because they believe. This is the operation of faith in action—when one believes they're becoming healthier as a result of trusting in pseudo-medicine. This is no more than what we often relate to as mind-over-matter. Mind-over-matter is nothing more than a level of consciousness or faith kicking-in commanding wholeness—to the body, mind or spirit. And thus, the statement holds true: *As a person believes in their heart/mind/spirit, so it is in their reality*. We can summon things into our reality with the proper perception—even when those "things" are not currently tangible. We have this incredible power to bring unseen things into the tangible realm simply by beckoning it. This belief is not only applicable to materialistic aspects but to the health of our bodies as well. I have personally been a practitioner of this concept for the majority of my adult life.

Living in good health as a senior citizen has become a common reality in many cultures around the world today. This is because many cultures are now placing emphasis on nurturing the *inner self* by thinking in terms of being whole. We see the practice of Tai Chi in countries like South Korea, Japan and China (before they banned it because of religious reasons). Tai Chi is a practice that involves a series of slow gentle movements and physical postures, a meditative state of mind, and controlled breathing. Tai Chi originally was for self-defense but evolved into a graceful form of exercise that's now used for stress reduction and to help with a variety of other health conditions. This form of exercise has even picked up popularity in the U.S. We see that people are living longer and healthier far into their senior years because of this paradigm shift in healthy thinking.

The body will become healed and whole when we focus our attention on being well and not sick. How many times have we encountered other people or maybe ourselves worrying about something to the point that we became physically ill? When all of the facts about the "thing" we were worrying about was revealed, we realized that the stress was unmerited. Too often, we manifest bad things into our own lives and blame the "devil" ..., and sometimes God—for being the source of our dilemmas. I believe that the fault lies within our own doings. We have not been fair to ourselves—for creating realities through our negative thoughts, verbal admissions and pessimistic anticipations.

In addition to creating good health through "right thinking," another applicable factor is being in harmony with our personal convictions. When we begin to create healthy bodies by correcting our thoughts and verbal admissions, we must not act in contradiction to what we know to do in the proper maintenance of the body. For example, if we believe that cigarette smoking causes lung cancer, but we continue to smoke thinking that our positive confession over our health is going to prevail, then we have "conflicting beliefs." These belief systems will clash, and one is going to be dominant over the other.

Conflicting beliefs will cause us to feel ill in our physical body—even though there is nothing physically wrong with us. When we neglect to take care of our bodies, i.e., by drinking excessively or smoking cigarettes, while expecting to be healthy—this is a contradiction. The two realities cannot exist at the same time in order to create a positive outcome. This is what I mean by conflicting beliefs. You will begin to feel guilty about being well when the other part of your psyche knows you're violating your own body. This guilt takes place on a subconscious level, and you may not even be aware of the internal conflict. Even though you are unaware of the conflict going on internally within you—it doesn't mean that you are unaffected by it—you are definitely being affected! When these negative emotions exist on the subconscious level, the creation will lean toward the unwanted manifestation of bad health. On a subconscious or (knowing) level, you suspect that cigarette smoking is doing your body harm, so the worst shows up, and your body manifests illness as a result of that belief. This is a very simple law—sometimes lost in the complexity of our rationalization. Many do not properly understand the dept that our emotions have in connection to belief. What we believe dictates our feelings, and what we feel can dictate our belief—depending upon which of them becomes the dominant focal point for you.

To live in divine health requires living in the awareness that good health is as much spiritual as it is natural. We cannot harbor bitterness, anger, hatred, vengeance, or any other ill emotion in our hearts and expect to live in optimum health. Alone with harboring negative emotions, our body's metabolism, hormones, and internal functions are affected by our emotions and moods. Have you ever noticed how those stressful situations will alter your ability to think clearly and function normally? Involuntary muscles, such as the intestines, which are responsible for breaking down food, can be affected by stress. The colon becomes sluggish and fails to properly break down the food— leading to constipation. This is because "colon motility" (the contraction of the colon muscles and the movement of its contents) is controlled by nerves, hormones, and impulses in the colon muscles. When the nerves, hormones, and electrical impulses are not functioning harmoniously—physiological balances get off, causing issues in the body. Stress hormones are also released into the body, causing unhealthy bodily functions. I don't want to sound too clinical—but our bodies will not function properly when our mind is heavy with concerns and stress. Our mind is the central control center for what the body does. So, if the mind is off-beat— the body will only follow the same off-beat rhythm.

So, it is clear to see how a good emotional state and healthy living are directly related to the proper nurturing of our *inner self* or spirit. We must be aware of our emotions at all times to ensure that they are in keeping and in harmony with our desire to be healthy and whole.

Think Healthy and Live Whole!

Article 17

Marriage Misconceptions

People seek marriage for various reasons but often fail to understand the underlining motives that lie deep within their subconscious as to why they want to be married. People usually feel that they are in love and believe that marriage will bring them the happiness or fulfillment that's missing from their lives. Most women marry for the sake of having that sense of security and the certainty of their mate's devotion. However, I believe that men tend to possess a sense of obligation that leads them to marriage rather than love. Now, this is not to say that men are shallow and do not possess deep caring love—because we do. But based on my observation of doing pre-marital counseling for many years, I believe that men commit to marriage out of a strong sense of responsibility and loyalty towards the woman. And for men, it is not usually the fluttering of butterflies in our stomachs that leads us into marriage. These feelings are usually associated to what women experience. Women are more emotionally connected to the whole marriage concept, whereas men are not so much. When I say women are more emotionally connected to the whole marriage concept—what I mean is that women think in terms of building a family. This starts with females at a young age when they're playing house, feeding, and tending to their dolls. A woman's need to be a nurturer begins as a little girl, while young boys, on the other hand, have no concept of family and being a nurturer because their main interests involve "roughhousing" and battling for dominance among their young male friends. But even though men's and women's motives for marriage might be different, there is still the need to be connected to another human being for companionship. This holds true for both men and women.

Happiness is still found in the differences between the sexes. But the first misconception that couples usually have is thinking that marriage is the fulfillment of their happiness. But *true happiness*, or, more accurately, "joy," originates from within an individual. Just for clarity—happiness is feelings brought about by good conditions such as getting a new car, house, a better job, or entering a new relationship. Happiness is conditional—but joy, on the other hand, is the state of mind or a state of "being whole" that is not dictated by circumstances. And often, for younger couples—marriage is expected to give them a sense of wholeness or completeness. But no one can create your sense of well-being because this is projected from your understanding of who you are. With this being said, in a perfect world, *wholeness* is what every individual should be bringing into their relationship. In the perfect world of relationships—both individuals are already possessing "joy." And joy is that sense of wholeness or completeness in one's self.

Another misconception is that marriage is the "cure-all" for loneliness. This, of course, is not true either—because some of the loneliest people I know are married. And being married, I can assure you that marriage often brings a shedding of friends—that can place you into a very isolating place. Your mate may not care for certain of your friends, and that relationship with that ole stand-by friend become distant. Your world of friendship can get a lot smaller depending on the insecurity of your mate. I am not by any means bashing or in opposition to marriage, but I feel that most people come into the marriage with their eyes "wide closed"—with unrealistic expectations.

I believe that most people do more planning for the wedding and place more emphasis on the wedding day than they do on the relationship itself. They then hope that the grandeur of the marriage ceremony will be reflected in the marriage. Many are *subconsciously* thinking that all the hard work for the relationship is over after the wedding. Planning a wedding and making it beautiful has nothing to do with planning your life together. There has to be a deep connection and compatibility in order for the relationship to endure the challenges that naturally come with being married. And with that being said, much of your hard work should take place during the dating period. This is when you determine your connectivity and compatibility with one another. And understand that connectivity and compatibility go much deeper than whether or not you like the same foods, movies, or activities. This connectivity and compatibility are found in the spiritual and intangible aspects of the individuals. A spiritual connection is basically a deep affinity felt between two individuals and goes beyond superficial personality traits, likes, dislikes, or shared interests. Instead, a spiritual connection is about sharing the same fundamental values, beliefs, life goals, and dreams as the other. And if these critical spiritual aspects are not in place, you will discover "real fast" how lonely marriage can be. So, marriage becoming the "cure-all" for loneliness is an unrealistic expectation—especially if the essential things mentioned are not in place.

The second marriage misconception is that being married will give you a sense of being complete. Marriage will not make you a complete and whole individual if you do not already possess a *level* of wholeness already. There are different levels of wholeness—and what most couples experience in the early stages of the dating process is usually excitement and infatuation. These feelings are often misinterpreted as feelings of wholeness. And for the record—wholeness is not a feeling, but is a state of being. It's a mindset that is not dictated by conditions. The excitement that a new relationship generates is simply the emotional effect of being a part of something new. In other words—it is no more than a new toy to play and entertain yourself with. And this is why after a little time passes—people become bored or uninterested in a partner—because the "newness" has worn off. They think that they've fallen out of love when in truth they've fallen out of infatuation. This sense of wholeness and completeness that one might experience initially in a marriage is typically short-lived after the excitement and emotion wear off. When enough time has passed, sex becomes a common act of duty, and the appreciation of the little charms fades away. The "real" aspects of marriage, then begins.

Often the "business" of being a husband or wife, a mother or father, becomes the priority of the relationship instead of the maintenance of romance. The "business" of who's going to pick up the children from school, what's going to be for dinner, what bills are going to be paid this week, and who's going to have time to help with the kids' homework—are just some of the issues that possibly stunt the romance. Though marriage is a beautiful institution, the maintenance of the family becomes the business aspect of the relationship that causes romance to sometime fade. And not only might the romance fade—but often, the feelings of incompatibilities and unfulfillment creep into the relationship because of all the responsibilities of managing a family.

I would like to mention one other aspect of being fulfilled that relates to understanding our individuality and knowing our individual needs. Too often, we expect our emotional needs to be met by our mates when actually the only person responsible for that need being met is you. People seldom get from their mates (or anyone else) what they really need emotionally—because no one at any given time truly knows what's in another person's heart in meeting that need. Only the one who has a need knows what is needed—and therefore has the responsibility of making themselves whole.

Being emotionally fulfilled is largely based upon one's relationship with *self* and not with one's mate. Another aspect of being fulfilled is personal growth which is also spiritual growth. When our lives reflect personal growth, we become more enlightened in our perception of life. We accept the responsibility of being in control of our own emotions and behaviors even when our mates do not satisfy our expectations. We will not harbor anger or regret or any ill feelings towards them when it seems that they are not contributing to our growth—because ultimately, it is not their job. This is not to say that your mate can't help or assist you in becoming all that you can be as an individual. But your individual growth is based upon your ability to mature spiritually—your ability to grow without the direct attention of others catering to you. No one can mature for you, just as no one can have your personal life experiences. Your spiritual growth is watered by your personal experiences, and it is a marriage misconception for you to think that your mate can spiritually mature you. Spiritual growth happens as a result of opening your mind to the unimaginable possibilities of the Universe expanding within you. However, your mate might be instrumental in helping you to become aware of the potential that lies within you—if they are consciously evolved themselves.

The last marriage misconception I would like to address is the belief that just because we are both Christian/ religious, there will be a mutual understanding of our spirituality. But being religious and being spiritual are two separate ideologies. *Religion can be defined as the belief in God or gods to be worshipped*—usually expressed in conduct and rituals such as belief, worship and etc., which often involves a code of ethics. Spirituality, on the other hand, can be defined as *The quality of being concerned with the human spirit or soul—opposed to prioritizing the material or physical things*. To put it plainly, religion is a set of beliefs and rituals that claim to get a person into the right relationship with God, and spirituality focuses on one's own feelings and convictions about what is right or wrong for them. Spirituality does not focus on doing good deeds to get to Heaven—because *spiritually* conscious people typically believe that Heaven is created here on earth by one's own perception. We should not allow religious belief systems, which are established by people having their own agenda and interpretations of truth—dictating what is best for us as it relates to our personal relationships. Every relationship has its own working dynamics when the two people come into that relationship whole and mature. They will be guided by their intuition (*the inner self*) in making the right decisions for their union. This is the importance of being whole when coming into a relationship.

If we obtain a sense of emotional maturity, it is usually due to inner growth that develops through life experiences. And because we are very resilient *beings*—when we face challenges in our relationships, we continue to thrive and grow. The challenges of unfulfilled expectations in relationships help us develop our sense of who we are. Our inner self and strength are fortified through our life challenges. In other words, we grow and mature when we don't always get things our way. And because of this, we put on our big boy or big girl pants, and we learn how to find happiness within ourselves. We don't require being coddled like a child when things become challenging in our relationship.

What marriage should be is two mature individuals understanding who they are and what they need, bringing their strengths together as a team. There should be an underlining purpose for the union if it is to endure the challenges found in every relationship. Marriage requires purpose to remain strong because where "purpose" is not understood, failure is inevitable. Every relationship that anticipates longevity should have intentions or an expected goal of accomplishment. There must be a common purpose to every meaningful relationship, including marriage, even as it is vital to have a meaningful goal and purpose in our individual lives.

Marriage should bring an increase of joy into one's life—but if you are happy, and spiritually fulfilled as a single person—then you would do well to stay single. Do not be influenced by others' expectations of you getting married just because you are of a certain age or because you haven't had children yet. Too often, we are made to feel guilty by friends and family if we are not in a serious relationship by a certain age. Parents expect us to give them grandchildren, and friends who are married expect us to join the "marriage club." Happiness and contentment are the best that life can offer any of us—and if you possess that as a single individual and feel complete without having a mate—then you are already whole as a human being. But the choice is yours, and no one can own your life but you.

Be Happy And Live Well!

Article 18

The Psychology of Men and Marriage
(Why do men marry?)

I have heard it stated by women who were in long-term relationships—how hard it was for them to get their men to commit to marriage. Being a man myself, it seems that we have a different perspective on marriage than women. I believe that some men see marriage as the ultimate gift that he can offer a woman—so some men save the marriage proposal the same way women *once* saved their virginity. Men typically delay marriage for as long as they can. And when many of us do make that marriage proposal—we often do so out of a rescue mentality. Men innately want to be the knight and shining armor that comes to rescue the damsel who is in distress. We pride ourselves on being the rescuers—saving women from the ideology that there are no more committed men. So, men will sometimes make that commitment to prove that we are exceptional—and in doing that, we become the knight and shining armor—and the king of the hill. Fairytale as it may seem—this is an unconscious response towards marriage for a lot of men.

If a man is tunneled vision in only what pleases his senses—he tends to commit to his pleasures rather than rationalization. What I mean is that he will only commit to a woman for the sake of having his senses and ego stroked. His motivation to marry is often fueled by the anticipation of being stimulated on a regular basis by the woman he deems to be the lady of our dreams. It is not always the overwhelming sense of love that men declare for women that lead them to matrimony. Of course, a man would never confess to that—but the need for constant physical, emotional, and ego stimulation is why I believe that men commit to marriage. I also believe this to be the same motivation for a man's tendency to cheat in a relationship. Because a man can always find at least sexual fulfillment from almost any woman if he is solely focused on being pleasured—even if the attention is only on a temporary basis. So, what marriage provides to the men who are knowingly or unknowingly looking for sexual pleasure *only*—are chasing an illusion of guaranteed ownership to sexual fulfillment. Unfortunately, it is not a realistic expectation because all relationships between men and women or otherwise will experience sexual excitement downtime. If his only goal is to be pleasured—without also considering her needs, then he has not developed a mature love—and therefore, is not marriage material. Neither has he come to understand the spiritual element of true love. This portrays the man who is immature and has not learned how to love—but is only pleasure-seeking.

However, this certainly does not ascribe that all men are immature because there are those of us who have the capacity to deeply love and to love maturely. But even those of us who do possess mature love—can too, have unrealistic expectations. Even "good guys" who are looking for true love—can show signs of insecurity and immaturity. These guys may have pure intentions towards women but constantly need their egos stroked. This is not a good look either for a man who is looking to be a husband. The "ego strokers" as I teasingly call them, are men who may have some underlining "mommy" issues. They need the "mommy figure" in their lives in order to feel a sense of value, worth and wholeness. This is often an unconscious need or expectation—but this kind of man may not be ready for marriage either, because his issues within himself are not resolved. He needs to become validated within himself first. And if he marries with this issue of needing constant validation unresolved—a woman is going to be dealing with what I call a big "man child" problem. He will require a lot of attention and securing like that of a temperamental child. He has not identified with the God source within himself that empowers him to be the confident man that a wife can confidently look up to. His woman will find herself spending too much time trying to grow him into the man she can emotionally and spiritually rely on. It also reveals that the little boy residing in him still desires to be the king of the hill. The little boy in him still needs the validation as a man—and this validation originates from the God source that should be emanating from him as an adult. Even with this flaw, he is capable of becoming a mature loving man if he is willing to expand his awareness of *self* by seeking knowledge of who he really is. But a conversion—or paradigm shift has to take place within him.

The understanding of who we are as men or as human beings directly effects how we see ourselves in a relationship. We must discover who we are so that we can be whole as an individual—therefore, being a whole and validated person in the relationship. We will then bring to the relationship a mature love for ourselves and possess realistic expectations from our mates. This mature love also brings a *whole* or mature man to the marriage. When a man is as whole and complete as he can be as an individual, he will then experience true love—the love that transcends to all of humanity and not only to his mate. He can be excited about marriage beyond the anticipation of sex. He can find that level of security he needs in one woman—because men, just like women, also marry for that sense of security—which is a basic human need.

As far as women are concerned (even though this article is focused on men), I believe most women tend to gravitate to the marriage concept more easily because of the mental programming that takes place in childhood—mental programming that is subconsciously actuated in young girls. Girls at an early age view marriage in a dreamier manner, whether the teaching of this view by their mothers is intentional or not. I am more inclined to believe that this perception towards marriage is simply innate to women. The mindset nonetheless, is passed down from mother to daughter, grandmother to granddaughter, or aunt to niece. Young girls witness the excitement found in conversations about marriage and the wedding dress, the ring, the flowers and so on. Because of this dreamy perception of marriage—little girls enjoy playing "House" and "Tea Time" or "Mommy & Daddy." So, at an early age, this dreamy occasion is constantly festering in their subconscious—making them more prone to this desire for matrimony, as I've mentioned in article 17, **Marriage Misconceptions**. We would probably not hear of a little boy wanting to play "House" with a set of dolls because boys aren't typically wired with this mindset. Instead, little boys are more drawn to "rough housing," wrestling, or playing games where they are competing to be on top or in charge—being the king of the hill.

When we see the dynamics of how young boys think and play—we clearly understand why men are not automatically dreamy about marriage. For men, there is usually an element of curiosity toward the woman that drives the desire for marriage. The kind of woman who creates excitement is the one who keeps us thinking and wondering about what's coming next. As men, we are motivated towards marriage when our women bring out that boyish excitement in us whenever we are in their company. This is the same enthusiasm we have as young boys when we are competing to be the king of the hill. Instead of being the king of the hill—the interest is now conquering the woman to make her our prize. So, when she becomes our prize, we began to want more for her than we want for ourselves. When our absence from her leaves us feeling empty or incomplete—we are in love. If a man has not reached that level of interest where he cares for his woman like he cares for himself, his love has not yet matured. When his care for her matures into love—he will water the garden of his relationship as he projects his own inner growth. To express the kind of care for another that takes a person beyond their own comfort is the manifestation of mature love. Mature love is what brings men to the possibilities of marriage. This kind of evolved love that causes men to love another human being as much as he does himself—and not just his woman—is what I speak of in article 19 entitled **Men & Mature Love** (*In the homophobic society.*)

There is a multiplicity of reasons as to why each man marries. Some marry because of sexual compatibility, or because the woman is a great cook, or because the woman shows great potential in being a good mother. And yet, all of the above could be the reasons. But nonetheless, we find our way to matrimony. We nurture our families and we water the garden of our love.

Men Do Love, and We Love Deeply!

Article 19

Men & Mature Love
(In the homophobic society)

In 2002 I moved from Nashville Tennessee to Atlanta Georgia. I became enchanted with Atlanta's beautiful skyline, and since most of my traveling to Atlanta was at night, the city always seems to be on display just for me. My work as a contracted electronic repair technician allotted me the opportunity to learn the city before actually moving here. The first place I fell in love with was Piedmont Park—being that I enjoy jogging and taking long peaceful walks in the park. But little did I know that it was a park where lots of gays/ homosexuals hung out. It is commonly known by most residences around the park, but unbeknown to me—that there is a designated area where gay men "hook-up." On this particular morning I went jogging at Piedmont Park when all of the sudden a guy came out and approached me with a proposition. I really didn't know that it was a proposition at first, because he spoke in a jargon that I wasn't familiar with. Because I was only interested in finishing my run, I dismissed him with the wave of my hand. But ten minutes later he showed up again on the trail, but this time blocking my path. The propositioning started once again—this time I got the message! I calmly told him that I was not gay and that I was a straight man. But he did not want to hear that and proceeded to grab me by my arm at which time it became a bloody fight. The police and the ambulance were called for an unconscious and bleeding man—needless to say that I was the conscious one who made the call.

I had never been homophobic or even knew that term before that experience. I had to go through a whole lot of self talk as to why "I" had to experience something like that—I felt so violated even though all the man got from me was a "beat down." At that time, I wanted to hate gays and homosexuals. But I could not, because I remembered what my parents taught me about excepting people who were different from me. I remembered what I taught my own son about accepting a world that has different values and beliefs from his own—so I found myself being true to my own convictions.

Our Western society today in 2021 has done a little better with accepting or either tolerating the LGBTQ/homosexual communities. I don't honestly believe that it has a mainstream of acceptance—because it is still quietly frowned upon. What's unfortunate is that our society is greatly homophobic. I say unfortunate because this suggests to me that people are afraid of those who have a different sexual orientation than their own. For a person to be afraid, intimidated or uncomfortable with another's sexual orientation, indicates that they are concerned with being infringed upon or either persuaded or simply uncomfortable. So, I am saying to my heterosexual brothers and sisters—

if we as heterosexual individuals (more pointedly men) are comfortable with who we are—then where's the threat? When I was approached at the park, I had no concern of being changed by another's anticipation—because I knew who I was and I more confidently know who I am now. The Piedmont Park encounter was a traumatic experience for me, but I yet understood that all homosexuals or people of the LGBTQ community are not aggressive and inconsiderate of others preferences. I have equally as much love for my gay and lesbian brothers and sisters as I do for my straight brothers and sisters. And though I am still evolving to a better "me," I recognize that my growth and maturity challenges me to accept all people.

When men evolve to a place of inner wholeness, our society will experience unity, peace and inner healing. Inner wholeness is the foundation, the birth place of mature love. I define mature love as loving without fear or reservation. Mature love accepts ALL people and is not govern by ego, nor is it concerned about being scrutinized or criticized while being friendly to the unpopular. Mature love embodies the belief of giving aid and comfort to the hurting without prejudice. Mature love is simply seeing and loving people the way God does—and if we want to know how God loves, just listen to our own hearts. Or either take in consideration how you would feel if someone chose to dislike you because of your race or ethnicity. Or what if you were snarled upon because of your level of education or the type of job you work. People have prejudices that have nothing to do with the quality of person you are. And without mature love governing our behaviors and interactions—we as heterosexual men cannot bring social healing to the straight or gay communities. This is not to suggest that heterosexual men (only) are responsible for making our community and society a better place in regards to accepting the differences of others sexual orientation. My objective in this article is to bring awareness to all men in taking leadership positions on making our communities a more accepting place for all people—gay or strait. And because the heterosexual community is still the majority in most places, we as the majority must be the leaders in reaching out to the minority groups and bring about more diversity & inclusion. My message here is not to change or persuade anyone of their sexual orientation, but to embrace one another as brothers and sisters—excepting the differences. And I'm focusing on the homosexual/ LGBTQ community in this article, because I know how contentious this subject is. We are not obligating ourselves to hanging-out or participating in other people lifestyles or activities—we are simply extending our hands of brotherhood by being accepting. We can live in harmony and yet have separate lives and sexual preferences.

When a man loves maturely, he is God-connected, loving himself and possessing a healthy sense of who he is as an individual. He becomes the embodiment of

God in male form, and he will serve humanity with passion and fervency. When a man loves maturely, he will water the gardens of his personal relationships with nurture and love, by giving the necessary attention to it. He never forsakes the sanctity of family. He is also able to show compassion to those of a different race, religion, ethnicity, social status or sexual orientation—because he realizes that his own son or daughter could become a part of a community of people that he doesn't personally prefer. The man who loves maturely has no preference to whom he shows kindness. The Bible states "*God gives his best—the sun to warm and the rain to nourish everyone regardless: the good and bad, the nice and nasty. If all you do is love the lovable, do you expect a bonus?*" (Mathew 5: 45-46 The Message Bible). All people are valued creations in the sight of God regardless of social status, race, education, religion or sexual orientation. I believe that all people are an expression of God. Yes…even the LGBTQ community!

Mature love does not choose who it will display itself to—for love is the nature of God as I stated in the beginning. God does not make a difference in providing for our human needs based on who we are—as we see in the Bible verse above. It does not matter to God if we are male or female, straight or gay, rich or poor, young or old, black or white—that determines God's provision. Because we are made in the image or from the spirit of God, we have the ability to love all human beings—to respond from a place of love to all humanity. When we as heterosexual men are able to love our gay and lesbian brothers and sisters—it is then evident that we are walking in wholeness and mature love. This not only applies to loving and respecting the LGBTQ community, but any group of people that we feel are unlike ourselves.

Are we able as men to display brotherly compassion to another male in a public setting? Or are we so egotistic that we become emotionally detached if we see the tears of a stranger who needs comforting in a public place? Are we able to avail ourselves to putting ourselves in someone else's position? It takes a spiritually evolved individual (or man) to portray brotherly-love to another man in a public setting. Will we become secure enough to embrace another male in a public place to give him comfort or encouragement knowing how our society might view two men embracing in public? These were some of the questions that I posed to 200 heterosexual men during a survey. I was greatly surprised by the responses I received because 178 heterosexual men out of 200 of them said yes—they would respond compassionately to another male in a public setting. So just maybe, most guys would be secure enough in their manhood to show this kind of public compassion to another man. And if so, I am grateful that this article is not implacable to most of us.

My real-life experience:

All of us can easily relate to consoling someone after loosing a loved one. But what if I change the dynamics of the story that went more like this: An obviously gay man in a hospital hallway crying inconsolably and it's only you (a straight man) and he, occupying this space. Because you make eye-contact with him—he expresses to you that his gay lover just died of AIDS. What do you do? How do you console him? Or do you even give him the attention that you would normally give anyone else? This was a very real scenario that I was once faced with about ten years ago at Piedmont Fayette Hospital. The gay gentleman was wearing these psychedelic rainbow bell bottom pants with platform shoes. It was obvious to me that he had been (or was going) to some type of 70ish costume party. I was honestly a little reluctant at first because of his flamboyancy and wild colors but then I looked passed his exterior and saw the brother's pain. His face was etched with hurt and his loud cries that eventually caught the attention of the nursing staff and visitors who were visiting their loved-one's—began to congregate into the hallway. I was deeply surprised...and hurt, that no one readily approached the man to comfort him. I knew their reluctance was because he was gay and flamboyantly dresses. But then I felt a deep pain of sorrow in my stomach...not because of the gay gentleman's loss—but because of my own shame I was feeling towards myself. It was as if I was under a microscope by the Universe questioning me," why *are you just standing they're*

131

like everyone else watching this man wail in agony?" In that moment, I remembered something my father once told me when I was a young boy. Daddy once said to me," *If you watch someone hurt another person, and do nothing about it, then you are no better than the one who caused the pain!"* Daddy was referring to a childhood fight where my friend got beat up, and was crying while everyone stood around laughing at him—myself included. I remembered how badly I felt afterwards. I felt so badly that I was unable to face my friend for a week. I dodged him for as long as I could until one day, he walked up to me while I was sitting on my porch. I was unaware of his presence at first. I will never forget how he looked directly into my eyes—and with hurt in his eyes, he asked me—*why didn't you say or do something—why didn't you stand up for me—I thought you were my friend?* I had never felt so much like a betrayer or a Judas Iscariot!

But coming back to myself in the hallway of Piedmont Hospital...I immediately went over to the sobbing gay man and without any words I gave him a deep embrace—pulling his head to my shoulders. I actually felt his body melt into mine in a sense of relief—the kind of relief that relayed—that someone cared enough about him to tend to his hurt, his pain and his loss. He embraced me back as if I was the only friend he had left in the world—all because I came over and showed him compassion.

That was the day I experienced a paradigm shift—I truly connected with the understanding of what it meant to love beyond your comfort zone. I also discovered that it is at times like this when we have the opportunity to serve as the comforting hand of God.

Public affection in other cultures:

In some African societies even today as an expression of friendship or honor towards a person—two men holding hands while walking down the streets is common. It does not signify that they are gay—simply a sign of friendship. When I was in South Korea in August 2010, I saw many business men in their expensive suits walking and holding one another hands as an expression of friendship. Sometimes they even held hands in groups of five while on their way to lunch. Because our Western society has such a misconception of masculinity, our heterosexual men suffer with male identity issues. Heterosexual men who do not understand what it means to be masculine often over-compensate their masculinity by projecting "hardness" or machismo. Little do they know that they are giving the impression to their young sons and other young boys who are observing the behavior that this is what it means to be a man. In actuality it is only teaching them how to be insecure and how to create facades. These young boys are only learning how to hide their compassion and to mask their insecurities. Many of these young boys come into manhood never learning how to verbalize their feeling of hurt or

133

anger—so they act-out as wounded misguided soldiers, devastating anyone who do not subject to their masquerade of insecurity.

It really doesn't matter whether you believe God to be an entity of compassion or not—because all you need to respond to—is the feeling of compassion in your own heart. And this is the same compassion that is in every human soul. If you will listen intently enough—you will hear the voice of compassion and empathy calling from deep within your *being*. This same voice is beseeching you to the action of empathy for your fellowman.

As mature men, let us walk as confident soldiers representing a compassionate Creator. Let us answer the call to action—to be the pace-setters for our neighborhoods, our communities, our nation—and ultimately the world. Let us show ourselves to be bigger than societies expectations.

Article 20

Homosexuals, Born or Made?

Because of the content of the material, I frequently write about relating to God or Higher Intelligence—I am often asked a series of questions concerning homosexuals. These questions consist of: "Are homosexuals born or self made?" What determines sexual orientation? What makes a person gay, lesbian, bisexual, or straight?

It has become obviously to me that these types of questions hold an undeniable interest to people in general. And I am keenly aware that these answers are still hotly debated both by the experts who study human behavior and genetics, the religious community—and by our society at large.

I interviewed and surveyed individuals of the LGBTQ communities about how or what introduced them to same sex relationships or same sex interests. What I gathered was a variety of stories that revealed to me that there are many dynamics to same sex relationships. However, I will state right off the bat that I do not have a conclusive answer—but I do hold the opinion that gays and lesbians (or non-straight individuals) are a combination of being self-made (by way choice)—while others I believe are born into it by way of genetics. A few of my gay friends expressed that they had experiences and influences that was in some form of sexual violation (at a young age) that traumatized and confused their sexual identity—that led them into same sex relationships.

In this article, I will share the information that I found in case studies that give validity to my opinion. I will also express my personal thoughts on the matter and share some stories given to me from individuals from the LGBTQ communities who identities are protected with fictitious names.

Biology and Sexual Orientation

Several years ago, I came across an article on Wikipedia entitled Biology and Sexual Orientation. This study deals with the research into the role of biology in the development of human sexual orientation. It is also stated that no simple, single cause for sexual orientation has been conclusively demonstrated. But research suggests that it is by a combination of genetic, hormonal, and environmental influences, with biological factors involving a complex interplay of genetic factors and the early uterine environment. Biological factors which may be related to the development of a heterosexual, homosexual, bisexual or asexual orientation include genes, prenatal hormones, and brain structure.

The majority of us have experienced sexual attraction toward another person, and when attraction is present it influences our behavior, mood, social interactions, and influences the image that we have of ourselves. Since this plays such a key role in our perception of *self*, it is only natural that we would be interested in knowing about its origins, and why we are oriented only toward people with certain characteristics and not others. Cristian C. Bodo in his August 7, 2007 article, Biology and Sexual Orientation states: "*Whether sexual orientation is the result of a conscious choice by the individual, as opposed to just another trait that comes "built-in"—will help determine if it should be categorized as a moral problem or not. This seems to matter a lot in shaping out attitudes toward sexual minorities. Specifically (for better or worse), the public appears to be more sympathetic to variations from the norm—in this case strict heterosexuality, if they are convinced that the individual has no authoritative opinion on this departure since it is the product of biological determination. On the other hand, sexual minorities have traditionally regarded this argument with suspicion. They fear that scientific research may open the door to treating these variations as little more than a disease and those efforts will be made to reduce or eliminate incidences of homosexuality in human populations.*" What I personally gather from Cristian Bodo statement is: In order for society to deem homosexuality as a moral issue, we must first determine the cause. What we believe about this matter will determine our attitudes towards people who are of different sexual orientation. People may be more sympathetic towards homosexuals if they view them as someone who has a disease or imbalance—not being able to control their preference. We must take into consideration that the LGBTQ community would not want to be viewed as being "sick" nor considered as being immoral. This diverse/ minority community would be treated as diseased individuals and being made to feel they were a lesser people—if we consider Cristian Bodo's assertion.

An experiment was done on male lab rats by castrating them at birth that showed that they no longer showed interest in the female rats after being castrated. The sexual drive for the male rats is induced by the testosterone hormones found in the testes. When the female rats were injected with the male hormone (testosterone) early in life, they later showed an attraction to other female rats. These experiments helped in the determination of sexual orientation. If homosexual tendencies are proven to be a disease or hormonal imbalance as we see in the experiment with the rats, how is it that we judge it as an immoral problem? As a society that frowns on illegal drug use, do we judge a new-born as immoral when they are born drug dependent because of a mother's addiction to drugs? How can the heterosexual society place judgment or deem those who are genetically or who are hormonally wired differently from us as being immoral.

Sexual abuse is another factor that could be responsible for those who are homosexual. As I mentioned earlier about a few of my gay associates…, this was their situation. And there is well-documented data that highlights that many (adult) homosexuals were sexually abused as children. The Associated Press noted in late 1998 that according to an analysis of 166 studies covering the years 1985-1997 as many as one in five boys were sexually abused. It also concluded that sexual abuse of boys is underreported and undertreated. It was also reported by a nationwide news media in May 2013 that numerous men in the military who are heterosexual, came forward and reported that they had been raped by other men in their unit. This act went unreported for years and is just now coming to surface.

Earlier studies have shown that 25 to 35 percent of girls are sexually abused before age fourteen. And if sexual abuse happens to a child that is one or two years old, he or she may not remember it later in life because it happened at such a young age. However, the trauma can still govern the psyche and affect the rest of the victim's life. Some homosexual men and lesbians will protest that they were never sexually abused, but if it happened in those earlier years that I spoke of, they might not have a way of recalling the incident/ violation.

However, there is another school of thought on homosexuals "not" being born with the same-sex orientation. The organization H.O.M.E. (Heterosexuals Organized for a Moral Environment) states: *"That there is currently no definitive proof that anyone is born homosexual. Several studies by homosexual researchers claimed to find some possible biological bases for homosexuality."* But other scientists easily pointed out the flaws in those studies, and the results of those studies have yet to be replicated by others. In the words of pro-homosexual **Newsweek** magazine: *"In the early 1990s, three highly publicized studies seemed to suggest that homosexuality's roots were genetic. More than five years later the data have never been replicated."* This fact has been almost totally ignored by the biased, untrustworthy, dominant liberal media. And in the May/June 2008 issue of **Psychology Today** stated: *"No one has yet identified a particular gay gene. There is no all-inclusive explanation for the variation in sexual orientation, at least none supported by actual evidence. There are many different mechanisms involving both nature and nurture, not a single one, for producing homosexuality."* This school of thought also believe that homosexuals were born heterosexual but experienced some type of sexual trauma that confused their sexual orientation. They also believe that homosexuals can be reconverted to their proper orientation. Yet another school of thought believe those who oppose using therapy to change homosexuals into heterosexuals, are in effect trying to keep homosexuals locked into homosexuality. Those who oppose such therapy do not want homosexuals to have a choice or a way out of homosexuality. This entire assumption and assertion is un-American, inhumane, intolerant, and meanly oppressive—argued by the organization H.O.M.E. Heterosexuals Organized for a Moral Environment.

However, I personally believe that there are those who are born with homosexual tendencies because I have personally encountered one-and-two-year-olds who mannerism was opposite of their gender. Before these children were of age to know anything about sexuality, they were portraying uncharacteristic behavior of their gender. One example of what I personally encountered was a five-year-old boy who favored wearing his big sisters clothing. The young boys' body movement and voice tone mirrored that of a young girl. His gestures were also quite feminine.

Another personal encounter was with a seven-year-old girl who was the daughter of a personal friend of mine. My friend's seven-year-old daughter preferred boy toys and preferred the activities usually only young boys enjoyed. In both of these cases, each child grew up being gay and lesbian—just as I expected they would. So, this is why I personally believe people can be born with an *altered* sexual orientation. And I use the term "altered" simply because their mannerism differed from their gender.

The question has been asked of me because of my personal assertion on the matter: *"If detected early by the child's behavior or genetic testing for dominant genes or hormone imbalances, can these children be treated with proper counseling or hormone injections?"* I am not an expert on genetics or hormone therapy—so I don't know. But my response is that in order to determine what should or shouldn't be done with young children who demonstrate certain gay or lesbian behaviors—allow me to first ask this question: Wouldn't it make sense to first identify if being gay or lesbian is a *true* abnormality? And if this condition is not a *true* abnormality, then there's nothing to treat. Could it be that this is simply something that we as a society are just uncomfortable with, so we deem it bad, evil, or immoral? I'm not pontificating that my assertions are correct, but I am deliberately challenging the perspectives that many have about homosexuality. I am challenging the reader to apply some common sense and critical thinking skills.

But what I do know with certainty is that no matter the person's sexual orientation, our basic human needs still remain the same. We all need love and respect, validation and security. The fundamentals of humanity should never be denied to anyone based on one's religion, beliefs, social status, race, education, or sexual orientation. I also believe that those who are prejudiced against the LGBTQ community are no different from the whites in America who supported slavery from 1776-1865. I clearly understand that this is a strong assertion to make—but the facts remain that abuse from authorities continued towards blacks during the 50s and 60s—and still today in 2023. And just as African Americans, and people of color in general—are still despised, hated, degraded, and are refused **certain unalienable rights** because of the color of their skin—this same hatred and prejudice exist among many towards the LGBTQ communities. Hatred, prejudices, impartialities, objectivity and etc..., are yet very real issues that we face as a nation and as a people. We are not a black race or a white race, nor are we a homosexual or heterosexual race—we are simply the human race. We are simply individuals either trying to find and make our way through life with as little conflict as possible. But homosexuals (nor any person) should ever be subjected to conform to a society that denounces their individuality for the mere comfort of the popular norms. All of us have a right to be who we are! Our constitution states: *We hold these truths to be self-evident, that all men are created equal, that they are endowed by their Creator with certain unalienable Rights, that among these are Life, Liberty, and the pursuit of Happiness.* **U.S. Declaration of Independence**

Same Sex Relationship Dynamics

These stories reflect some of the relationship dynamics that I mentioned at the beginning of this article and how some were introduced to homosexuality. Their names have been changed to protect their identity.

Bob, a 36-year-old gay man, tells his story of how when he was 9 years old was taken into a church closet by his Sunday school teacher on a Saturday evening after a church event and was molested. He was told by this adult Sunday school teacher that if he told anyone, the same would be done to his younger brother, who was only 6 years old at the time. To protect his younger brother, Bob kept quiet about the matter for two years—the entire period that this violation went on. But little did Bob know at the time that the same Sunday school teacher had already been molesting his younger brother, who was given the same threat. Bob expressed to me that he had never had any desire for boys before this experience—in fact, he had a girlfriend when all of this first happened. When he turned fourteen, Bob had his first voluntary sexual encounter with a male who was four years older than him. From that point on, Bob seeks out men for companionship even though he is still attracted to women and dates them. Bob's younger brother also turned to men as a teenager, and neither of them knew of the other lifestyle until years later into adulthood. Because of social pressures and family, Bob had to keep his sexual orientation a secret, so in an attempt to *denounce* his lifestyle, he married a woman that he was deeply in love with. That marriage lasted twelve years, but Bob still had an attraction to men.

Sylvia, a 26-year-old lesbian, had her first sexual encounter with a girl when she was only eight. Sylvia always knew that she had an attraction to girls, more than she did to boys. She stated that she remembers kissing other little girls on the lips around the age of 4 years old and would get spankings regularly for it. She did, however, date and have sex with men but found it uncomfortable and unsatisfying. Sylvia says that she has never been sexually violated but has always had a desire for the same sex.

Lou, a 40-year-old male/transvestite who was molested by two of his uncles from the age of twelve to seventeen, enjoys sex with both men and women. Lou prefers sex with women more than men but likes to dress as a woman when "picking up" women. Lou stated that his uncles chose to molest him and not his two younger brothers because he (Lou) would entice his two uncles. Lou's two younger brothers had very feminine characteristics, and Lou was the masculine of the three, but it was Lou who considered himself "freaky," as he called it. His brothers have never been in any same-sex practices, and furthermore, both of Lou's brothers became the "ladies' man" when they reached their early twenties. These same brothers are both in successful marriages and feel that Lou's lifestyle as a transvestite is repulsive.

Cindy is a very attractive 32-year-old woman with two young boys. She was introduced to lesbianism out of a game of "dare" at the age of eighteen. She states that when she became a young adult—she found herself being curious about having sex with other women, but wasn't particularly attracted to women sexually. She stated that after five years of "only satisfying her curiosity" by experimenting between women and men—that she became hooked on having sex with women. I asked Cindy, "What was it that hooked you into this attraction with other women?" She told me that it just felt more natural for her to be with women than with men. But Cindy stated that when she wants to feel safe and protected, she prefers the company of a man. Cindy has a ten-year-old son, but only allows her son to see her with her male companions because she feels that this is the healthier perspective of a family. Nevertheless, she states that: *"I must have my girlfriends on the side, and I will never marry a man."*

Terrance and David are two middle age homosexual men who had both been married to women in their past lives. Currently, they are living as gay lovers on the "down low" or the "DL," as it is commonly called. This couple has been in a relationship and living together for more than twelve years but states that they will never get married. They stated, *"Marriage between two people of the same sex is an abomination to God, but cohabitating is acceptable*." While other gay unions are fighting for marital rights, Terrance and David totally reject the idea of marital rights for gay couples and live their lives quietly and discreetly.

We can clearly see the many spectrums of perceptions in same-sex relationships. What I have learned is that people have a variety of sexual appetites and tendencies that is too complex to judge. I do not know who possesses the authority to deem homosexuality an immoral act or sin—or if it's indeed a moral or sinful issue at all. Could it simply be that this is just another God-given choice or experience to this thing we call life?

Just as children are born into the world with deformities, couldn't homosexuals also be born with sexual tendencies that they are pre-exposed to genetically? Some religious people might say that God cannot make a mistake that would cause them to be homosexual or lesbian—but isn't it strange that when a child is born with one arm or no legs, we do not challenge God on an error made? If we believe that God allows some children to be born with (what we perceive as human beings—seeing that we have limited knowledge) a handicap—who can say that homosexuals are not in the same category? Who can deem that any so-called birth deformity is a mistake? Since we are human beings with limited understanding and insight, we cannot completely know what the mind or intention of God is. Therefore, we cannot rightly

147

judge a birth defect, whether it is physical or genetic, as an error or mistake. We would have to be the creator of the creation in order to distinguish the purpose and functionality of the handiwork. Therefore, we should never proclaim to know the path that any life should take—except our own.

Though I truly believe human beings to be God incarnated, I am also persuaded in my own heart that our humanity sometimes prevents us from understanding issues like this clearly. Therefore, let us not seek an occasion to be offended by others' sexual orientations. Our *higher self*—where I believe God dwells within us, leads us as human beings to not judge this matter and these individual situations from our human perspective—but to simply show compassion and love to all mankind as our main objective.

Let us only be concerned about loving and healing the spirit of humanity by allowing every individual to have their own life experiences—understanding that we are not the determiner of the path, that others choose to take.

Article 21

Married, But Attracted to Someone Else?

In a world of imperfection (at least from human perspectives), I find it interesting when people look for perfection in marriage. Most people's definition or understanding of what a perfect relationship consists of is unrealistic. Most people hope that their marriage will be without personal conflicts—even though we understand that to be unrealistic. We do not anticipate that there will be challenges with old or new attractions. But as "real-life" would have it—these things often come up. And the failure to understand that there will always be distractions (other people that you're physically attracted to) will be one of your gravest misconceptions.

As human beings who innately desire new experiences and new adventures, we will meet other people while in a relationship that will also attract our attention. It does not mean that we're in pursuit of someone else or have intentions of being unfaithful. But it does showcase the curiosity that we possess as human beings and our attraction to variety.

Most people who have been in long-term commitments have had previous relationships. And sometimes past relationships can undoubtedly smear over into current ones. These feelings and attractions from the past can still exist between people who are no longer together. And emotional ties do not necessarily go away just because you are in a relationship with someone new. Instead, these ties can lie dormant in the realm of our emotions—sometimes undetected until later. Often, we don't even recognize an interest until we see an *old flame*. Seeing a former partner in a grocery store that you hadn't seen for years can drum-up old feelings. Even a particular song on the radio or a scent of cologne or perfume can stir up old feelings and memories. Often these experiences are innocently and unexpectedly encountered. And with certainty, these old emotions can and usually do surface at some point in a relationship that often lie undetected or hidden within a person.

Undetected and, in some cases, unsettled emotions from past love relationships often do not show up until problems arise in the current relationship. It is when things go wrong in the relationship i.e., lack of attention shown, or loss of attraction, or simply boredom—that these occasions of reminiscence of a former relationship creeps in. Sometimes in marriage, we become bored and lose interest in doing new and creative things with our mates. And not necessarily because of any conflict between the two—but simply what I refer to as relationship complacency. This complacency is a level of comfort whereby people fail to see the importance of actively putting in the effort of keeping the relationship alive. When this complacency happens—people will often find their minds or heart wandering in another direction from their mates. This when people find themselves slipping back into old attractions from their past while being married. And this same relationship complacency can open up the door of curiosity with a completely new person… i.e., someone from the job. This is why it is imperative that we keep things exciting in our relationships. See Article 23, **Why People Cheat in Relationships** & Article 24, **Oatmeal Sex…**

People enjoy new relationships because of the excitement that comes from learning and experiencing something or someone they've never known before. That whole "getting to know someone" process is stimulating to our senses. But often in marriage, life between two people becomes complacent and predictable, and the marriage goes down the long unwanted road of boredom. Many people in this marriage situation began to seek out someone to share some fun conversation with—but too often, that fun conversation leads to spending fun time together. And it may not necessarily be with the intention to *physically* cheat—but the so-called harmless flirting can get us into some big trouble if we do not stay in check of where our emotions are trying to carry us. But when you play the flirting game too long, you'll find yourself on a wave that is too strong to swim out of. At this point, a person's heart no longer belongs *completely* to their mate. They have become distracted.

When we allow ourselves to be *wooed* into a relationship outside of our committed relationship—this becomes an usurpation of the ego. This is true for both men and women. And yes, this is only the actuation of the ego. It is not love but infatuation that's birth from the desires of the ego. This dichotomy, unfortunately, happens more often in relationships than what many would confess to. However, I am not advocating that anyone would go outside their marriage or monogamous relationship just because they get bored or become unsatisfied. Nor am I advocating that people allow exes back into their lives (or anyone else), when they are in a current relationship. But let's not be naïve in thinking that we are immune to innocent flirting—which can lead to the whole snowball effect of infidelity. And though you may deeply love your mate—you can be pulled into an attraction with someone you initially meant to be platonic with.

Yet, there are some cases where you might find yourself *actually* in love with someone who isn't your mate. It could simply be a case of still being in love with someone from your past. But I am here to tell you that there are many people who are married wishing they could be with the one that they truly feel connected to—and yet remain faithful and loving to the one that they are committed to. Like the song Luther

Vandross sang, "*If you can't be with the one you love, then love the one that you're with.*" Lots of people are doing it every day! It is the unfortunate reality that sometimes shows up when real-life happens.

Expiration date on relationships:

I personally believe that relationships have an expiration date—particularly romantic relationships. And what I mean by having an expiration date is to say that relationships become familiar, predictable, boring, uneventful, and simply stale like old bread. The fact is—this is to be expected. If you ride your favorite amusement ride a hundred times, it will eventually lose its thrill. But just because your relationship becomes stale doesn't mean there's no value left in it. Even stale bread is useful in making stuffing, chicken batter, croutons, and a crispy topping for a casserole—so there is still potential in that ole bread. Our relationships can become very much like stale bread—though it may not have the same appeal, freshness, or *newness*, there can still be an appreciation for it. Your mate may have gained some extra weight, loss hair, grown a few wrinkles, lack in energy, complained more than before and the list could go on. But keep in mind that you have changed too! This is the time when we reevaluate "what we do have" in our partner. Perhaps the predictability is the result of someone who cares enough for you that they "endured" your changes to become that familiar with you. And maybe things becoming boring and uneventful are the result of you

153

giving up on finding new and interesting this to do with your mate. And just maybe, your complaining mate is crying out for the attention and the small considerations that you once gave. Relationships do not simply become stale because of time—they become stale because the individuals stop doing the things they did when they first met. Often couples stop trying to impress one another after a period of time with the misconception that it is no longer necessary to put that much energy and effort into the relationship. And like stale bread—we have to recycle, reconstitute and revive the old relationship. And this takes a lot of physical and mental work!

Most people who are married aren't living their fairy-tale life with their fairy-tale mate—but that doesn't mean that we can't still have a marriage full of excitement and adventure. Create an adventure in your relationship by first appreciating the person that you have. Express to your mate that you still appreciate them—and you will nurture to life the creativity and bliss that you thought was lost. We need only to possess a realistic view of our humanity and understand that Higher Intelligence is always guiding us into optimum maturity.

Love yourself... love the one you are with... and watch your relationship grow into a masterpiece.

Article 22

Do Opposites Attract?

At a meet-up group in Atlanta, Georgia called "Battle of the Sexes" or B.O.T.S. as we nicknamed it—we held a spirited discussion as to whether opposites attract in relationships. We typically think that two people have to have the same likes and dislikes in order to have a harmonious relationship—at least, that was the general consensus of most in the meet-up group.

But when I think of attraction in relation to people, I automatically think of the dynamics of how magnets work. I think of magnets because in order for a magnet to attract to another magnet, the north and south poles have to face one another. In other words, if the two north poles of the magnets are facing one another—the magnets will push away from each other. So, it takes a negative and positive (a north and south) pole in order for there to be a connection of forces. And I believe the same is true when it comes to people attracting to one another. Let's look at the meaning of the word "attract,"—which means *to cause to come to a place or participation in a venture by offering something of interest, favorable conditions, or opportunities*—is one definition. According to Webster's New World Dictionary, it means to draw someone or something to itself. So, in relevant terms, it means to cause someone to have a liking or interest in you. In a relationship, to attract is the same, which means to *draw to one's self, to adhere to* —but I would like to add that it also means *to be in harmony with or connected to*—just like in the example of the magnets. If we can focus on the definition *of being in harmony*, I believe that it will lend us the clearest understanding of "attraction" as it relates to relationships.

When we are in harmony with another person, we feel a sense of connection—a sense of oneness or a feeling of agreement. We have heard the saying, "birds of a feather flock together." This saying stems from a belief that people tend to associate or *draw to, adhere to,* or *be in harmony with* those who are like themselves. But let's keep in mind that we are as much spiritual beings as we are physical beings—and that we also connect on a *spiritual* level. An elementary example of having a spiritual encounter with someone is when you meet a person for the first time, and right away, you sense a "like" or "dislike" for a person without even knowing their name. It is like we become in-tuned to an aspect of them where we're able to determine a certain familiarity (or not) with them. And this sense of familiarity can either feel positive or negative. What we are actually experiencing is conscious connection or disconnection (depending on the experience). Again, this is retrospective to the positive and negative forces between the magnets.

So, when we're attracted to a person (or them to us), we are simply sharing harmonious energy with that aspect of them that is akin to our desire. This is to say that we draw the type of person whose attributes are closely aligned to our own. Consider this query; why does the quiet, conservative man find himself drawn to the boisterous, outgoing woman? Most of us might think that they would have nothing in common. But could it be that the quiet man sees in the boisterous woman a quality that he wishes to possess? Could it be that his attraction to her is because, subconsciously, he desires to be more outgoing like her? So, he finds himself attracted (or draws into his realty) someone he can vicariously live his unexpressed desires through. I have experienced this in my own life. I do not consider myself to be a good dancer and wouldn't risk the embarrassment of dancing in public—but I found myself drawn to women who are great dancers, who love and is comfortable dancing in front of others. With her out-going personality, I now find the confidence that I have always longed for—to also dance with groups of people. And even when I'm standing on the sidelines watching her—I am vicariously dancing in the company of others through her. She is able to express a part of me that I am too shy about expressing in front of others. So, my attraction to someone who appears to be the opposite of me (at least in this regard) ended-up being the hidden expression of me. The attention that I secretly desired—is now expressed through her.

Just as we attract the person who's able to express and bring out our inhibited side—we can also attract someone who might bring out an aspect of ourselves that we don't want people to see. Our inhibited side could also include a "dark side" to our character. This is why we must be careful about who we allow ourselves to become attracted to. Neither should we allow people into our life who are semblances of what we're trying to avoid. For example, if we no longer entertain drinking alcohol because of some substance abuse issues from our past—we would need to be very intentional about "not" linking up with someone who is involved in that life. We may find that we are still attracted to a certain behavior or conduct because of our familiarity with it. But if this is what we are trying to avoid—going forward, we must circumvent the exposure of ourselves to this energy.

Years ago, we used the term in church, *kindred spirit* or *a familiar spirit*. These terms indicate a "soul-tie" that could become the catalyst for entrapping someone into a relationship or situation that was once escaped. It was commonly understood in our religious community that it was vitally important for us to steer away from people that had *kindred* and *familiar spirits* (energies) with. Mainly, if those energies of familiarity had negative influences. To this day, I carry this belief in my heart even though I do not consider myself a religious person. But the principal of this concept, I yet find to be sound and true. It is of great importance in understanding what is drawing us to a person beyond their physical appearance. We must be sure that we are not drawn to them because of our attraction to old habits. And not being intentional about the creation of the relationships that we draw into our reality—is why some people end-up in situations that they don't want. These bad situations include abusive relationships, toxic lifestyles, debt, depression, unfulfillment and a host of other unwanted situations.

Why would the *abused* attract an *abuser* into their life? This is a good question to ask because most people would not purposely invite someone into their life who is abusive. Unfortunately, many people unknowingly attract abusive relationships and situations into their reality. They have no clue why the situations they've been trying to avoid keep showing up in their lives. They are creating their realities by default—meaning not being deliberate, precise, or conscientious about where they are giving their creative focus. Read article 10, **Overcoming Abuses**.

Ultimately, we draw or attract those who are in synergy with us. The subconscious attraction we mentioned a moment ago derives from the core of our being. This is the same energy that we display to the world as confidence or weakness, joyfulness or sadness, wholeness or neediness, love or hate. Whatever energy we project to the world or people around us—will by that same energy attract into our reality. One who focuses on their abuse, pain, or anger will attract into their life those very things. And the same is true for the one who focuses on finding peace, love, and harmony will also attract the same into their life. So, whatever you give your attention to is what will boomerang back to you. Therefore, we must anticipate meeting people who are emotionally and spiritually healthy for us. And those healthy relationships will become our reality as long as we remain focus on that. The same is true when we anticipate or expect negative people or situations to show up in our lives—they also manifest. Our emotions are tools or magnets for attraction. We simply attract what we give the most attention and energy to.

Lastly, keep in mind that we will only attract that which resonates from within us. We have been given by Higher Intelligence the ability to summon the unseen to the seen, the intangible to the tangible, and the supernatural to the natural. All of us possess the creative ability to form the realities we wish to have. So be conscientious and deliberate in what you allow yourself to be attracted to.

Article 23

Why People Cheat in Relationships

Both males and females share the same basic need in relationships, and when these needs are not met, some people tend to search for a sense of fulfillment elsewhere. In surveying 100 men and women who had cheated in past relationships, 75% did not intend to be unfaithful—they were only interested in having a new experience with a new person that did not necessarily involve having sex. It started out as harmless flirting with no other intentions. And many of these individuals who took this survey expressed that they simply wanted a little extra attention that involved compliments and the sharing of time. Both men and women in this survey stated they felt that their partners, mates, or lovers seemed uninterested in them—so they sought someone who could fill that emotional gap. Many of these individuals even expressed that they were not particularly physically attracted to the people they flirted with. They simply like the feeling they experienced when they attention was shined upon them. They conveyed that they deeply loved and cared for their mates. Taking into consideration what this survey revealed, there are three key points I would like to make concerning the misconceptions about people who cheat—and they are:

1. People only cheat to get extra sex on the side.
2. Once a cheater…always a cheater.
3. If a person is unfulfilled in a relationship—they are going to cheat.

Depending on one's *inner constitution* or personal *convictions*, cheating may never occur during the relationship, regardless of personal dissatisfaction with the relationship. I find that the motivations of every individual who does cheat are surrounded by a different series of interests for cheating. And I will go back to each one of these three misconceptions in detail further into this article. But I feel it's necessary at this point to establish the foundation of what keeps a relationship solid and harmonious before going any further. Because of the dynamics of relationships, it's imperative to stress what is needed in a healthy relationship in order to prevent the potential deterioration that leads to infidelity.

As I mentioned earlier, males and females have the same basic need in relationships. The first fundamental element of a healthy relationship is respect. To feel respected is to have a sense of honor and value bestowed upon you—this is how the ego in every person is stimulated. The ego, or one's *image of self*, is what primarily governs about 65% to 75% of our actions and responses in our relationships—and in every other aspect of our life. When we feel devalued or unappreciated by our mates, it can sever the cord of romance and destroy sexual attraction as well as any other attraction that we have towards our partner. Even in the midst of disagreements, respecting your mate's feelings and showing sensitivity will fortify the relationship bond. But if you do the opposite and call your mate out of their name during a disagreement, you will weaken, if not destroy, the relationship bond. The people we love must feel valued at all times—and all the more when there is friction between us.

This is why name-calling should be eliminated in arguments—because once you *release* those words into the ears of your mate, you cannot take them back. And those words can scar and possibly destroy your partners' image of themselves. And it can be hard restoring a person's *self-image* after shattering them with a degrading remark. Even when an apology is later given, a person may still remain wounded. Reconciliation on the *soul* level is not easily made once a person is wounded.

The next fundamental element of a healthy relationship as it relates to *the self-image* is telling your mate how attracted you are to them. Everyone's body changes over time, and none of us are going to remain in our twenty-year-old bodies. It is so crucial that we continue to admire and regularly flirt with our mates. People like to know that they are still appealing in the eyes of their lover—and even to others. I believe that when someone harmlessly flirts with us by way of a compliment, meaning (flirting without any intentions) is healthy for a persons' self-image/ ego. When you deny your mate the attention that they deserve by not flirting or complimenting them—it can become the basis for them stepping out of the relationship. This is not to say that we are solely responsible if our mate cheats on us if we do not give them enough attention, but we can, at best—do our part in securing our mate's egos.

Now let's begin addressing categorically the three misconceptions about people who cheat. In reference to misconception number one (1)—People do not always cheat just to get extra sex on the side: Often, it is a matter of getting attention from others who build their self-image and make them feel good about themselves. As I stated earlier, sometimes, it is simply the attention that is not being received from home. No matter how long you have been with your mate, they need to hear you say, "*You still turn me on*,"—and it should not only be said when sex is wanted (referring to the guys). If you do not remind your mate of how attracted you are to them, someone else will certainly express their attraction to your mate. This is such a major component because our sexuality and sensuality are intertwined with our *image of self* or the ego.

Misconception number two (2)— "Once a cheater…always a cheater" is another misconception. There are many dynamics as to why people cheat. Granted, some cheatings are premeditated, but others might be an unexpected encounter that is introduced by finding yourself in a compromising situation. It makes no difference as to how one is trapped in a web of infidelity—cheating is not necessarily a compulsion for everyone. Some "step out" because of lack of personal attention given by a mate, as I mentioned earlier—but as I've heard many people say—they cheat in order to get even with a cheating partner—which I've never understood since the objective in cheating is not to get caught. So, I do not understand how one is getting "even" if the other is not supposed to know about it? Still, others may become temporarily bored sexually with their partner or may need validation in regards to feeling attractive and "still having it." Others may simply "step out" out of mere curiosity about being with someone new. No matter the reason, it does not mean that a person is going to do it again. How many of us have experimented with drugs and alcohol or gambled away our hard-earned money? Maybe we did these things only once—or let's say we've done them a few times. But nonetheless, we stepped away from doing those things and never returned to it again. Well, someone having an affair can be exactly the same—just a "fling." And please understand that I am not trivializing an affair by any means—but the point I'm conveying is that, as human beings we are highly sexually driven creatures—coupled with curiosity. And sometimes we faulter in our commitments. But I would be remiss in adding that once a person cheats and gets away with it, it does become easier to do it again. The excitement that comes with experiencing a new adventure with another person is a human dynamic—that is propelling.

For some people, their *image of self* or ego is directly connected to their sexual abilities. What I mean is that some people's (particularly men but not exclusively) value is in their ability to be a good lover—so they participate in every sexual encounter they can find. They are promiscuous—and they convince themselves to be the best. This is commonly termed as being "whorish,"—and this person could be a man or woman. And if we are referring to a man who commits to this behavior, he's the guy with a boyish mentality wanting to be the "king of the hill"—who's still attempting to conquer the prize. He is slaying the dragons of his sexual desires—but does not understand that he is a man who is unconsciously searching for his identity. I talk about this more in-depth in article 18, **The Psychology of Men and Marriage** (*Why do men marry*).

And when we are referring to a woman who's exhibiting this promiscuous behavior—she is conveying the girl who is seeking the approval of a father or to gain control that lends her a semblance of protection and security. This may be reflected in the absence of security or control as a child—a child that might have experienced some type of physical, sexual, or emotional abuse. So, she frequently engages in

166

affairs to gain the attention/ protection that she missed as a child. And yet, she may simply possess an insatiable appetite for sex. This, again, could be true for either men or women. Nonetheless, either of these individuals craves the ability to conquer by having multiple sexual partners because, on some level, this behavior defines their self-worth. And as unnerving as it may be—infidelity becomes commonplace for people with these issues.

Unfortunately, cheating, in part, is the complexity of many relationship issues. It is a common reality. But I am by no means condoning or advocating cheating in any relationship for any reason. I believe that there is enough relationship diversity in the world today to not have to cheat, i.e., "swingers." Swingers are those couples who invite other couples or individuals into their bedroom—giving themselves sexual diversities. If you are a person who likes having sex with multiple partners but yet feel the need to have one person that you're committed to in a relationship—this lifestyle might be for you. But my advice is to find someone who shares your belief and perspectives on the matter. And do not violate the sanctity of a relationship by getting with someone who believes in monogamy. And let me say for the record—that I am neither an advocate of having multiple sexual partners, because I understand the psychological, spiritual and potentially physical degradation that this can have on a person's life.

I have learned that human nature will always rise no matter what your religious affiliation is. I know parishioners who experienced "fleeting affairs." I have been told confidentially by some of these individuals who had engaged in an affair—that had they not found a sexual out-let at a crucial point in their marriage—they would not have had the fortitude to stay married. They stated that they would have ended up in divorce if they didn't have an affair as a buffer. I know this may sound a little crazy—but this is where people are. And no one is excluded from potentially falling into these situations—because I personally knew these parishioners (both men and women). These same men & women have now been married for many years and are yet with their spouses, but they stated that they have never had an affair since. Some people have fleeting sexual experiences to simply get through a rough patch in their relationship—not necessarily always looking for a way out. It also does not mean that they are settled on making cheating a habit. Once again, I am not advocating infidelity in any situation, and by no means am I making light of this potentially hurting act, but simply stating that cheating is prevalent. It is simply the unfortunate reality of human behavior in many relationships.

Let's look at misconception number three (3). Anyone who is unfulfilled in a relationship will cheat: Even though most people become unfaithful because of a lack of fulfillment (in whatever area of unfulfillment), it doesn't necessarily mean that they will cheat. Some people have very strong convictions about remaining loyal and faithful in relationships. Some are faithful and loyal, even to the point of totally sacrificing their own happiness to remain true to their mate. These people live with a heightened awareness of observing personal morals and high values. Their ego or *image of self* is often defined and validated by their ability to maintain a clean and clear conscious—which is admirable. Living in a mindset of self-respect and self-honor is their mission. The comfort that they find in remaining faithful in an unfulfilling relationship—is the same thing that gives them their inner contentment. Their contentment stems from their observation of keeping their marital vows. This lends to a higher level of self-confidence and dignity—and they find solace in living with integrity. Needless to say, they observe a high constitution and are a rare breed.

And yet there are others who remain true to their relationship regardless of being unfulfilled—for the simple reason of not jeopardizing losing their family if they were to get caught. They simply stay faithful for fear of the risk in losing their family.

A lack of fulfillment does not equal a cheating mate, but in our relationships, we should always do our best to be the best mate we can be. We should always consider the needs of our partner as we consider our own. Give your partner the love and attention that you would give to yourself. Your partner will hopefully see your efforts and reciprocate that same affection.

Article 24

Oatmeal Sex... B-o-r-i-n-g!

Sex is to be enjoyed by both parties, and this act of expression needs a little variety every now and then. Some men and women feel that the mere act of having sex with their mate is enough to sustain the satisfaction—but that's a huge misconception. I believe that variety is indeed the spice of life. A change in position, experimenting in various places, and even a little role-playing might be necessary every once in a while, to keep the lovemaking experience fresh and new. Ignore the bedroom creativity—and you will end up with "oatmeal sex." Oatmeal sex is boring sex—the worse kind of all, because it lends to bedroom complacency. The relation I am making between oatmeal and sex is that you can eat oatmeal every day, for the remainder of your life, and it will nutritionally supply your need. But how starved would your taste buds be? Well, the same is true about boring sex—it might knock the sexual edge off, but how dissatisfied will your sexual taste buds be?

Many people are starving for the sexual excitement and ecstasy that should be found in their relationship. But their sexual experience is just enough to knock that sexual edge off—but not enough to satisfy the deep longing for true sexual connection. Many couples rely on their partners to tell them that a change is needed in the bedroom. Often, the concern of hurting the partners' feelings prevents this needed communication from happening. But in order for sex to become exuberating—serious and open dialogue needs to happen. The open and honest communication of what's needed or expected must be expressed. But this conversation has to be handled with sensitivity and consideration. But if your partner doesn't know what is needed or expected—no change will take place. And if a couple wait to see if things will magically work itself out—without talking about it—you will be fooling yourselves—and you will end-up with "oatmeal sex."

From years of serving as a marriage counselor, I have observed that many problems in relationships are issues relating to sex. Probably more vocalized by men because men are usually more focused on physical pleasure, as I stated earlier in article 18, **The Psychology of Men and Marriage**. And the women in these counseling sessions and those who participated in the group studies I hosted—were a little more reserved about this issue as it related to their men. And what I noticed about the women who had very little to say about their husband's sexual short-comings in the bedroom—was that if women were overall pleased with the way they were being treated in the relationship—did not speak negatively about their men. But they did express, in general, the desire for their men to engage in more foreplay and creativity.

Typically, women are more focused on the security that their men give them—which adds to a woman's sexual satisfaction. But if a man fails to secure his woman by not taking the time to fulfill her emotional needs—she will likely begin to feel neglected. Consequently, when a man thinks that sex is all about him and is only interested in his needs being fulfilled—it becomes a sure recipe for bedroom and relationship disaster. And this, without a doubt, will cause women to feel neglected faster than anything else. And when women are made to feel unappreciated and devalued—especially in the bedroom—they will become very vocal about the man's inadequacies. She will burn every listening ear about his bedroom short-comings. This is simply a woman's way of expressing her frustration—and her cry for attention. And guys—if your woman is on this merry-go-round of frustration—you better hope she doesn't find another guy to vent your short-comings to—because this could lead her to cheating.

When a person is left unfulfilled in the bedroom—they will become *emotionally naked*—or commonly termed, vulnerable. Keep in mind, that both men and women's security lie in the consideration that is given to them from their partner. And let me also add that it's imperative that couples have the freedom to verbally expresses what their bedroom needs are. Sometimes we don't always know what our partner need from us in the bedroom at any given time. Because of the everyday stresses of life—both men and women—physical and emotional needs can frequently change. And so, it's no wonder that sexual performance, can and will become an issue at different times in a relationship. And by the way—this happens in every relationship—no matter the orientation of the relationship. The business of simply living sometimes interrupts peoples' interests in sex—and they become what I call, "bedroom complacent."

But we cannot allow this kind of complacency to settle in our relationships—because couples can become tempted to cheat. Not because they have fallen out of love—but because they have fallen out of excitement with their mate. If *physical* cheating does not become an issue—individuals find other means to cure their sexual frustrations by flirting on the job or online, turning to porn, or masturbation. Couples must find ways to bring a little "kinky" back into the bedroom.

Lend to your partner whatever is needed in the bedroom (within reason). Respect each other's needs—and do not be judgmental of your partner's sexual cravings. Just as people have different food preferences, they also have different sexual preferences. Your partner should not be judged as immoral just because they enjoy "kinky sex" and you prefer conservative sex. People's appetites for sex change in relationships, even as our appetites for food changes as we go through various phases of our life.

The one who likes bananas is no more, or any less normal, than a person who likes peaches. This is also applicable to our sexual preferences and appetites.

We are ever-growing and ever-changing beings in every capacity of our humanity—including our sex lives. So, add some spice in the bedroom and throw out that boring "Oatmeal Sex."

Article 25

A Relationship Issue
(My Friends are My Friends)

How often have we heard of couples getting into arguments about one another's friends or complaints about how the other spends too much time hanging out with old acquaintances. How do we handle it when this "hanging out" with friends consists of ex-boyfriends or ex-girlfriends? And should we denounce our friendships with all exes? This is a very common feud that we hear about in almost every couple's relationship at one time or another. And though this issue is not regularly discussed between couples because there is usually an unspoken understanding that all exes are not to be entertained anymore—people often secretly hold on to exes as platonic friends. So, the question that I've been posed with is—should we automatically discard our exes as platonic friends, when we come into new relationships?

Right off the bat, this is a conversation for individuals who have an open and mature *sense of self.* First, we must look at the two individuals coming into the relationship. It is important that we understand who we are as individuals. If your mate is naturally jealous of "anyone" who occupies your time—then you may have an overly sensitive partner. And in this case, you need to abandon all communication with an ex for the preservation and out of respect for your relationship. If you understand that your partner has the propensity to be excessively jealous—you should consider your mate's feelings and not try and convince them to get over an ex that you are declaring to be platonic friend. A person whom we might consider as being overly jealous may have had a heart-breaking experience, and now they're unable to trust freely. We cannot change people because we are not able to undo the experiences that have shaped them into who they are. This is why it's vitally important to take the time to know and study the person we are getting ourselves involved with— before committing to a relationship.

On the other hand, there are several situations with people that I know personally who are in committed relationships and yet have exes that are still platonic friends. In fact, the exes in some of these cases—hang out with the couple on social occasions like sporting events, birthday parties, baby showers, and holidays. And for all intent and purpose—things seem to be quite harmonious. I've seen where the exes actually became friends with their exes' mate. Now I am acutely aware that this doesn't (and won't) fit into most couples' agreement—but I feel that it's worth mentioning that there are many who manage these unique dynamics.

So, we must understand that in some relationships, exes are allowed—when they can be trusted by remaining platonic and posing no threat to the relationship. However, there has to be a mutual agreement and a lot of open and honest dialogue between a couple. Ground rules have to be specific and clear. And to protect against any potential *old feelings* creeping up—there should be an understanding in place that no alone time with an ex will be permitted. I personally feel that a REAL friend (whether ex or otherwise) will never jeopardize your relationship—and if a person attempts to violate or disrespect your union—it's time to dismiss them from the circle.

Our mates should always encourage healthy friendships because we all need those special people in our lives that motivate and inspire us to reach our optimum potential in life. Sometimes as much as we love and appreciate our significant others, they may not necessarily inspire us. Sometimes the people closest to us can become our worst critics, and at times we need a break from them. But having that go-to person in your corner can enhance your life. We should not be obligated to forsake meaningful and healthy relationships with old friends if they bring value to our relationships by making us better people. This might mean that a spouse or mate may not care for your friend, but this friend brings the best out of you. As a mate, you may need to take a back seat and allow your partner to maintain that friendship. We are not obligated to like or prefer the people whom our partner deem best for us. We are individuals with independent needs, and it's okay to have a separate group of friends from our mates. Again, as I said in the beginning—this conversation is for mature and level-headed thinkers.

It is my opinion that human beings were not created to be owned by one another but to co-exist in harmony and in liberation. This is to say that any relationship, which imposes emotional or physical bondage on a person, is not giving value to individual wholeness. In a relationship, we do not own the other person's *individuality*. People must be given room to possess their values, uniqueness, and their friends without infringements upon those rights. Liberation is an expression of the presence of God's spirit. True love for our mate will allow us to release that person to have their friends (who bring out their best). But each person in the relationship must know whether they can handle having a separate group of friends in a relationship—especially if this friend is an ex. The relative questions to ask are:

1. Will having a separate group of friends from my mate be an issue for them?

2. Can I be content with my mate spending time with my group of friends who might consist of an ex?

If you cannot answer "yes" to both questions, this would be a good place to start communicating your expectations and establishing boundaries for your friendships. These are the imperative conversations people need to have in the dating process.

Article 26

Maintaining Your Identity
(Don't Loose Yourself in Relationships)

When we think of identity, we may ponder the question in our heads, "who am I?" But who we are is found in the composition of the experiences that have molded us into what we present to the world as "I." We also embody the collection of beliefs about one's self. We generally take a lot of pride in who we are as individuals and what we've become. Our identity of *self* is tied to the accomplishments and failures that we have made throughout our lives. Our self-esteem and ego are intertwined and sometimes consumed by how we are viewed by others and how much we are respected by the people we love. Everything that encompasses us—helps us to identify, or at least gives us a perspective about who we are and how we are viewed by others. Our self-esteem is heightened when we feel admired by our friends and family—knowing that our life means something to someone else. We relish in our identity.

Three questions you might be asking—the first one is: How do we lose our identity in a relationship? The second is: What happens when we lose our individuality or identity in a relationship? And thirdly, how do we get our identity back? These are the questions that I'll be addressing a little later in this article.

I will first begin by explaining the dynamics that surrounds the affects of giving too much of ourselves. People have the tendency to give more of themselves in relationships than what they're *consciously* willing to give. After giving so much of their love, affection, resources, time, and attention, some may feel a sense of regret afterward if their giving goes unreciprocated. When a person gives of themselves in a relationship, and it is unreciprocated (or given back in kind), they often begin to feel devalued. An aspect of our human need is to feel valued and accepted, and when what we give is perceived as not being appreciated or accepted, we feel rejected. And when we encounter what we perceive as rejection—we will begin to lose a sense of personal identity in that relationship. We may see ourselves as not being good enough or feel unappreciated. As I stated in the beginning, that part of our identity is connected to how we are perceived by the people we love. Often women are the victims of this dichotomy because of the nurturing character that women innately possess—their need to be a *giver* to the ones they love.

If a person gives of themselves and feel that they are not equally reciprocated—they will begin feeling bitter and regretting that they have given so much of themselves. At this point, one might feel devalued. And people in general, do not feel good about themselves when their efforts of trying to please goes unrecognized. This can often be interpreted as the *receiver* being ungrateful—especially if the *giver* fails to understand that reciprocation is different from person to person. Human nature is motivated through recognition.

To address the first question at the beginning of this article: How do we lose our identity in a relationship? To answer succinctly, we lose our identity when we give too much of ourselves. What I mean is that when one gives so much of his/ her time, attention, sex, gifts, or availability—and it begins to feel laborious, emotionally and physically draining—that is usually a sign that you are over-giving. Giving should always be organic and feel authentic. And let me also add—that when we begin to *unrealistically* expect others to give back to us in the same manner that we gave to them—we set ourselves up for disappointment. We should never do *tit for tat* (equivalent given in return) because each of us possesses a different set of value systems that governs how we respond. Our different value systems (things we hold or esteem highly) will vary depending on our frame of reference or experiences. An example of having different value systems is when a man shows his love for a woman by being the best provider he can be. This might entail the man working long hours to provide her with the things she wants. On the other hand, a woman might show her love to a man by showing him affection, cooking a special meal, or maybe doing something as simple as running errands for him. Both individuals are expressing their love for one another, however different it may be, and though the actions are different, the expression of their love for one another is equally genuine. Men and women—and people alike simply give of themselves differently. We cannot determine for someone else how they should show their love and appreciation for us. Every individual uniquely expresses themselves the way that they do.

Now addressing the second question: What happens when we lose our individuality or identity in a relationship? I actually touched on that when I mentioned earlier that people (men & women alike) become bitter, angry, or resentful towards the other person when they lose their identity in a relationship. When a person gives of themselves in a relationship, and it is unreciprocated (or given back in kind), they often begin to feel devalued.

In answering the third question: How do we get our identity back? You should stop giving more of yourselves than you're willing lose—because you are truly "giving away" a part of yourself. This simply means to stop giving with the expectations of a return. Do not give until you feel emotionally bankrupt or until you feel regretful for what you've given. And when you stop doing these things mentioned—you will begin to feel empowered once again. Your *sense of self* will be restored because you now have reserved energy, time, and attention to yourself.

Giving of ourselves only as it feels comfortable— will prevent us from experiencing that sense of "losing ourselves" to another—or losing our personal identity. We maintain the constancy of who we are as an individual when we stay connected to our own needs and desires.

As we regain our personal identity—we must also recognize our uniqueness and our value as an individual. We can celebrate who we are as a human being because we are unique within ourselves. This self-awareness is crucial because if we fail to possess this healthy sense of *self*—our self-value or self-esteem will diminish—resulting in a feeling of unworthiness. It will serve us well to remember—not to allow ourselves to be imposed upon. Give only what you can as feel authentic to you—whether it's your time, attention, finances, or love. We must take back the power of our identity by being a little selfish— meaning having a sense of one's self or needs, as I related in article 12, **Why Should I Be Selfish**.

Lastly, do not imprison your identity to your job, cars, houses, financial status, or anything of the sort— because materialistic things will never define the true essence of your *being*. You are uniquely and wonderfully made!

Article 27

Compatibility & Love

There are various aspects of compatibility and love that must be addressed in order to gain an understanding about the importance of the two. The first thing we must do is to define what compatibility is and the common errors people make in confusing it with love. They are two separate aspects with very distinct differences.

Often people think of compatibility as liking the same foods and enjoying the same activities. While these things are important in a relationship—however, it does not define what compatibility is. So, let's start here with its definition: Compatibility is defined as mutuality, being in harmony with, well-matched, suitable, or to be congruous. Compatibility is the fundamental nature of having common interests or needs. All healthy relationships must have a common interest, a common fundamental belief system, and mutual expectations in order for the relationship to thrive.

Compatibility in its purest sense connects individuals on a deeper emotional and spiritual level. When people truly experience compatibility—they feel like they are being heard, seen and cared for when in one another's company. There is the comfort of safety in being able to let "your hair down," with the freedom to be your authentic-self. True compatibility allows deep engaging conversations to happen without the fear of ridicule or judgement. The conversation is easy and transparent—and there's no need to wear a façade. When you are compatible with someone, you enjoy their company and look forward to the time you share together. And it feels like there's not enough time in a day to spend together when you feel this type of connection with someone you are compatible with.

I know that in the beginning of most relationships—it feels like all of the above splendors mentioned. And sometimes we mistaken compatibility for love. But you can actually be in love with someone and not be compatible with them. Because the true essence of love has nothing to do with feelings—but has everything to do with commitment and action. Allow me to explain by first define the meaning of love. True love is a unique and passionate bond that connects you to another person and it causes you to want the best for them—even at the expense of sacrificing your own desire. True love does not keep a score of all the wrongs or faults of another—it looks for reasons to forgive when offended. True love does not lurk around corners—waiting to see if someone is going to make a mistake. Love will prevent a mistake from happening—because its nature is to protect. And I could go on with countless example and expression in defining love—but I think you get the message.

Both love and compatibility are very important ingredients for a healthy relationship. But is there one that's more important to focus on when searching for a mate? I think there is!

From my personal experiences and failed relationships, I am inclined to believe that compatibility is the most important element when considering a mate. The issue I discovered in my past failed relationships, was that I *did not* or *could not* find a place of compromise in our expectations of one another. Our core values and core convictions did not line up so that we could fulfill one another's expectations in the relationship. No matter how much we loved each other, we found ourselves struggling to get along—consequently, becoming frustrated in our efforts—we finally grew apart. I know there's validity to this point because when I held couple's discussion groups, I realized that many of their issues—and failed relationships had also stemmed from incompatibilities in one area or another.

Determining compatibility with another person involves time in getting to know a person from the inside out. And this is where compatibility is often missed because people tend to establish romance before establishing true friendship. They allow themselves to develop feelings before determining compatibility. They feel that just because they have *things in common* that they know enough about one another. But having common interests with a person does not necessarily equate to being compatible with them. Having things in common, like enjoying the same foods or movies, liking the same colors, and enjoying the same activities…just to name a few—will not equate to longevity in a relationship. Of course, all of those things are good, and it is great having someone who shares similar interests—but neither does it equate to compatibility.

Compatibility also involves a connection on a spiritual level (that I will address at the end of this article) and not just the superficial things I mentioned above. But within the friendship stage, you come to understand one another likes and dislikes—and it is during this time that you see whether there is compatibility. We experience freedom when we are not required to alter who we are just to be with someone. The sense of being one's self lends to the foundation of a good relationship. This is why I believe that the friendship stage is so important because it allows us to grow unrestricted or confined to the norms and expectations of a romantic relationship.

The factors that make us compatible shines a light on what our core needs and convictions are. And our convictions encompass the contents of who we are on a spiritual level and reveals the essence of our belief system. And our belief system is rooted in our influences and becomes the guiding force for our perception of the world. This integration is what teaches us how to function in a relationship—and how to be civil in the world around us. Without sounding too technical—my point is simply: when seeking a mate—slow it down and get to know the true heart and soul of a person before you allow yourself to fall in love. Take the time to find out if they are a spiritual or religious person, if you are seeking a relationship for longevity. This is a huge factor that should not be overlooked if spirituality/ religion is important to you—because it is easier to fall in love with someone whom you share deep spiritual/ religious values with.

In my closing comments—if you are seeking someone to grow old with—do not invest your time romantically until you are certain about compatibility. Romantic involvements creates a deep bond that can give a false reality of being in love. So do not rush into romance because this could turn into a trap for the desperate-hearted. The possibility of finding love will always be available in various stages of your life. But falling in love with someone that you are incompatible with can be a huge trap for yourself—because it becomes hard to separate yourself once love sets in. I believe that it is easier to love someone you are compatible with than to "become" compatible with someone you love. Think about that statement for a moment! If you find yourself in love with someone but later realize that you are not compatible—you will not be able to break away from them because too much of your heart has become invested. And though you may continue as a couple—you will find it quite difficult to enjoy everyday life because of the differences over what's essential. Being in love with someone that you are not compatible with will become a tumultuous relationship.

Falling in love should be the most natural act for a human being. So let us not put so much effort into trying to find love—rather seek compatibility. Allow love to find you—and in the meantime…, love yourself.

Love will always follow friendship, and friendship will always harness love—for it is easier to love someone you are compatible with than to "become" compatible with someone you love.

J. Meddling

Article 28

Perception Transference
(I am not "You")

Have you ever encountered that person who thinks they have the answers to everybody's solution? That person on your job who think they know more than their boss—or who think they could run the owner's company better than the owner themselves? Or, how about that person who proposes their opinions—and who tries to subject everyone else to it. They act as if the sun rises and sets on their every command and that the world would be a better place if everyone thought like them. But I guess if we would be honest with ourselves—we all have moments when we feel that way. Sometimes, we simply want things to go the way we them to.

It's not as much to deal with when you have the occasional "know-it-all" to contend with—but what if you had to be in a relationship with a person like this? What if you had to wake up every morning to a person who was always asserting their opinion on things? That relationship would get old pretty fast! Well let's not pretend any longer—you are in a committed relationship with Mr. or Mrs. "know-it-all" or…, "it's my way or the highway."

I have given a term to the people who value and usurp their opinions and beliefs over everyone else's— I call it **perception transference**. This behavior is undergirded by insecurities and control. Both behaviors are indicative of one another. But the continuous *pushing* or insisting on possessing the same interests, affiliations, and preferences that I relate to as perception transference—has to be managed. All of us, from the time-to-time struggle with the differences that we have with other people—but in general, most of us understand that our differences should not be superimposed upon another. And the reality is—we as individuals are not the same. We have different values, beliefs, opinions and perceptions. I am not you…, and you are not me.

Sadly, many potentially good relationships have a person in it that feel the need to usurp their views on the other. We do not have to see everything through the same lenes as our partner in order to have a harmonious relationship—but we do have to respect one another's views and perspectives if we want harmony. Granted, it makes things so much easier when we are in a relationship with someone whom we share things in common—but when one person attempts to transfer their beliefs, habits, or lifestyle upon another, based upon their own perception—it becomes problematic. And this kind of control can lead into a behavior that lends to suspicion that is concocted in a person's mind. Let me give you a real example from my personal experience. Years ago, I had a friend who became romantically interested in me, but because I never made advancements on her, she assumed I was gay. I did not understand why she felt that way about me, seeing that we only considered ourselves friends—so I felt no reason to cross the "romantic line" with her. She had known me for several years and had always known me to be a "straight" guy. *But then I reflected on something she shared with me about herself. She had "experimented" with being in a relationship with a woman years prior to meeting me. I remember her explaining that this relationship with the woman was only an experimentation with her sexuality. She was trying to **find herself**—as she stated. However, she did not consider herself a lesbian just because she was going through an experimental stage with a woman.* I began to connect the dots to her past when she told me that she knew that she was an attractive woman—in which she was—and that any man who wasn't interested in her would have to either be gay or was trying to figure out his sexuality. As a result of her past experience, and because I showed no romantic interest in her—she felt that I was going through an experimental stage with my sexuality, just as she went through years earlier. **Now…, how messed up is that!** Needless to say, I was so a little taken back when I understood that she was relating my sexual orientation to her own past experience. Though she may not have been conscientious that she was projecting her experience on me—I clearly understood what was happening. And since that experience—I have encountered and identified many cases where people are operating out of this behavior. And sometimes it's a matter of people wanting you to have the same weaknesses and disparities as them—so that they don't appear as being less than you.

And for the sake of not appearing to be less than you—these individuals believe that if they struggle with something—you too must also struggle with it. This is why I believe that people who have cheated in relationships—as well as those who are "cheated on"—find it difficult to trust a partner's faithfulness. And they become suspicious of others in the same matters that they've been guilty of. This not only applies to cheating—but to something as simple as keeping promises. If you often break promises or have had promises broken to you—you might have a hard time believing that others will keep the promises they make. This mentality can be portrayed in any area of our life where a person is insecure with themselves. As I stated in the beginning, the root of this issue is often insecurity and the need to control. Again, both behaviors are indicative of one another. And the saying that misery loves company—does have validity. But this is what perception transference looks like.

A person's perception can be misconstrued and lead to the devastation of a relationship. The wrong perception can destroy a potentially good and healthy relationship. Therefore, we must come to appreciate the differences and opinions of others and accept one another as we are. But making this conversion takes a certain amount of discipline to release our ways, beliefs, opinions and perceptions to allow room for someone else's. We must discipline ourselves to see the good and the value of living in a diversified world—and not subject others to our own perception. We must see that people are potentially good regardless of their differences from our own. We must understand that others experiences have molded their beliefs—just as your experiences have formed your view of the world.

People impose their fears, likes & dislikes, beliefs and perception onto others—not necessarily because they want to—but in most cases because they do not recognize the trap that life experiences have placed on them. They function and operate as robots that are being controlled by a remote user. And in this case the remote user is their subconscious. Years of misinformation, bad experiences and emotional trauma is often the precursor to their problem. And somewhere along the road of life, they have forgotten that we are their comrades—soldiers in the same battle of life. Worn and beaten as they might be—these people have their place in society too. We are the human race—though we hold separate opinions and beliefs—we are all fighting on the same team in life.

I am not you—and you are not me, but we are all part of this wonderful universe where we were meant to live by the support of one another through the power of Higher Intelligence. Let us live, laugh and respect the differences of one another. Let us awaken to the reality, that we are all one—created equally but as individuals.

Article 29

Life after Disappointments

Like a boxer who is disoriented by a punch, "takes a knee," or a time-out to reestablish his senses—we too must take a time-out to regain our senses after facing disappointments in life. Various life situations can give us a crushing blow. And no matter how much we pray and believe, we will always have to deal with the jolts of life. But I believe it would be helpful if we would learn to see disappointments as a vehicle that brings us to a deeper awareness of *self*. People seldom practice self-evaluation when all is going well—just like the boxer who sees no need to take a time-out when he is winning the fight. But on a continuous basis, we should evaluate where we are emotionally, physically, and spiritually. Focusing on being and feeling complete is the emotional and mental space where we need to be when facing life's disappointments. If we can master staying in this mindset of being a winner in life—the effects of life's disappointments will be minimized. The Universe is always in constant communication with our *inner self* or spirit—but failing to take the time to quiet our spirit and center ourselves causes us to miss the divine instructions that come from within. These instructions are critical when facing the challenges life throws at us.

Disappointment comes in every form imaginable, but some can be more devastating than others—especially in the case of a loss of a loved one or a break-up from a relationship. And the reason these two forms of losses hit us so hard is that much of our *self-identity* is wrapped up in them. We are innately dependent upon one another for physical, emotional, and spiritual survival. Our need for one another is part of a survival mechanism placed into the threads of our humanity. People define who they are by the relationships they establish. We feel good about ourselves when we are surrounded by people who validate our worth. But no matter how protective our friends and loved ones are of us, they cannot protect us from the disappointments of life. And just because we get knocked down in the first round of life does not mean that the fight is over. How many times have we seen a boxer gets knocked down in the early rounds of a fight—only to see that fighter recompose himself to win the fight later? Life is no different. It is simply a matter of understanding that in life, there will be many challenges and battles to win. When we understand that we have been prepared and conditioned from birth for this life that entails struggles—we can then draw from that assurance that we can and will recover from every challenge.

The key to overcoming disappointments is to not focus or give attention to where you are in the present—but focus on your anticipated future, just like any professional athlete who visualizes a successful win before the competition begins. Therefore, we cannot focus on past mistakes, misfortunes, or losses—because that will impair our vision of crossing the finish line. This is not to say that we should not take time to grieve a loss—nor negate the time of recovery from a blow that life gives. It is only natural that we give a healthy amount of space to process what we're feeling at any given time—in any given situation. But we must, at some point, get through the grieving period, the stagnation or frustration—and move our thoughts, attention, and actions forward. We must strive to get to a better emotional space—that place of feeling whole and complete. Whatever ill emotion you're dealing with, whether it's feelings of anger, hurt, rejection or etc., they're all feelings of disappointment. Focus on the good that you wish to feel—in any given situation, and you will multiply positive emotions—that ultimately bring positive manifestations. You will become a testament to yourself that you can overcome every disappointment. More importantly, you are a co-creator with the Universe that works through and with you—to make your life what you choose it to be. So, recompose yourself—push straight ahead and continue your fight.

Article 30

The Rejection Games

Experiencing rejection in a relationship can feel traumatic—causing us to feel abandoned and lost. We have seen how people try and hang onto failing relationships—even when the other person has emotionally moved on. And often, the rejected person already knew that the other person had been looking for a way out of the relationship. Still, the rejected person strives to salvage a dying or dead interest. And how about when the person you are pursuing rejects you—and you finally move on—only to discover that they are now interested in you? And in the opposite, when we encounter someone who's interested in dating us—but we have no interest in them—but as soon as our pursuer moves on to someone else (because we showed no interest)—suddenly we become interested in them. It appears as a game of cat-and-mouse where you make an approach to capture, only to have something evade you. These are the facets of what I call the Rejection Games!

It is complex how we as human beings develop an interest in people or things after forfeiting them. This gives insight into our psyche of how greedy or protective we can become when giving up something or someone we really have no interest in. I do not believe that we consciously play this game, but it is innate to our human characteristics. I learned from many years in sales that if you want to get a customer hooked on a product before actually selling it to them—it is important to give the customer a sense of ownership of the product. This is achieved by having them to handle the product, test drive it, taste or smell it, or to try it on for size. Whatever it took to make the customer feel a sense of ownership is what we did as salesmen. Creating a sense of ownership is what stimulates the human ego to possess. Once we test drive the car that appeals to us—we gain a sense of ownership—and there's no way we can leave that car on the lot for someone else to drive home. This same dichotomy takes place when we experience a buffet of people to choose from in the dating game.

Sometimes people can act psychotic. And I say this because—we pursue people that we want—and we even want those whom we've rejected. We especially see this happening when we suddenly desire to be with someone we previously rejected—all because we perceive that someone else was interested in them. We then want "ownership" as if they are a piece of property! We become covetous of things and people we don't "really" want—but for fear of losing them to someone else—we try and hoard them like a possession. Doesn't this mirror psychotic behavior? It is definitely Dr. Jekyll and Mr. Hyde conduct. And maybe all of us have a little of this "craziness" in certain situations. But this kind of behavior as a way of living, can be detrimental when exhibited in a relationship. People with the mentality of *possessing* another—can become abusive when they are unwilling to let-go of a relationship. I am not necessarily speaking of being physically abusive—but abusive in the sense of being controlling. This type of control can become mentally and emotionally devastating for the other person. This is representative of the insecurity that one carries—that feed into their need to *possess* or *own* someone as if they are property. And this is considered abusive behavior. It is the need to maintain a *sense* of ownership that drives a person with this mentality. In this case, the fear of *loss* paralyzes the one who is unable to release someone they are not really interested in. But the fear of giving up someone with the possibility of someone else having what you really don't want—is a definite sign of a person with a control issue. Insecurity and control are only a couple of factors in the rejection game.

This rejection game has a variety of dynamics that might not be considered. For example, there are people who fear rejection so badly that if they sense the other person is about to break-up with them—they will create disharmony to initiate a breakup. Again, this is the fear and/or insecurity of them having to be the initiator so that they won't appear to be the lesser authority in the relationship. This is also a control factor that's being displayed. They need to be in charge and in control of the direction of the relationship at all times. This is the same scenario that is played by an employee when a boss tells them that "You're fired," but the employee responds by saying, "You can't fire me because I quit!" This is simply the ego saying that *I will have the upper hand*—and *I will have the last say*.

As human beings—we do not like excepting no's or being denied. But this is because we were created in the image or likeness of Higher Intelligence. We are internally wired to divide and conquer and our drive for life is insatiable. So, when we are forced to face rejection, we quickly and yet unconsciously go into protection mode. We protect and defend the aspect of ourselves that is tied to the ego. This protection sometimes resembles the attitude of "*I don't care*" or "*I can take you or leave you*" mentality. But the ego puts on facades when facing rejection—and the "*I can take it or leave it*" mentality is nothing more than the ego trying to "*save face.*" People will often say after being rejected that "*I'm really all right...*" when on the inside they feel emotionally tortured. And though it is in our *God nature* to be winners—we must also understand that we are not entitled to the dismissal of real-life experiences. Rejection is simply an aspect of our human experience.

Unfortunately, rejection is a painful part of our humanity, and we must always be aware that we are not responsible for being everything someone else wants. People will make choices to except us…, or not.

Therefore, rejection will be a part of our reality. We must understand that it is not our responsibility to try and control the decisions of others by manipulation, fear, deception, or force. And lastly, let's hold our heads up high as we realize that we are the most powerful force to be reckoned with on the earth. And because we will face rejections in life—let's keep in mind that our destiny yet lie within our own hands and not in the disappointments we face in life. So, let's keep our lives moving!

Article 31

Understanding the Role of People in Your Life

In order to live intentional or purposefully—we must have an understanding of why we've chosen the people in our life. When I was in sales—our team manager had a saying that I will never forget. He would say…, *You will only go as far in life as the people you associate with.* And at twenty-two years old I understood the value of having quality friends and associates. Four years later I was introduced to a European business mogul name Terry Hansen. Four eight years I traveled around the world with Terry learning and observing how to conduct business with millionaires. What I learned in those eight years set the course for the rest of my life. And the business practices I learned—I applied to my own life. I have been in business as a self-employed individual for more than twenty-five years. I have owned and operated multiple businesses in various industries.

For me, it is clear that our association is a crucial factor as to how far we go in life. Who we choose as friends will significantly determine our quality of life. So, I have adopted a saying that states: *"I am only as whole as the circle is around me."* And too often (like pieces on a chess board), we attempt to place people where we want them in our lives. Of course, there is nothing wrong with strategizing or organizing the placement of people in our life as to deem their value to us. But when your friends/ associates try and manage for you their placement in your life—it can become problematic. We have all experienced having that person who deemed themselves as your best friend—when in reality you only saw them as an associate. And there is a huge difference in having a friend and an associate. A friend is someone who is down for you in your darkest hours—an associate is someone who's cool to hang-out with every now and then—but not someone whom you engaged into your affairs. But sometimes people see themselves more valuable to you, than you see them.

If you're to have social structure—you must understand the roles people play in your life.

I personally have four categories that I place people in—and though everyone has a role to play—only two of these categories are essential.

1. **The Convenient Role** is usually something that just works well for everyone in involved. I typically classify these people as associates—and I call them when I'm interested in going to a music festival at a park. They are someone I want for casual/ non-personal company. I won't typically engage in deep or lengthy conversations

with them. These are the people that I only choose to participate with when I feel like being bothered with them. It's not necessarily me being selfish—it is just something that naturally works out.

2. **The Situational Role** is usually my co-workers or colleagues. If there's a work meeting or a function where we are all called together to brainstorm a work project. And I might even hang with them out-side of work to gather information from them because of their expertise in an area. I classify these people as associates.

3. **The Obligatory Role** would include my family—because these relationships I classify as essential because you don't choose your family—we are simply born into them. I have siblings that I dearly love, but some of them I would not have as a friend if I knew them in another capacity. And if you feel pressured to get along with anyone—be it family or not—it might be an obligatory relationship.

4. **The Ride or Die Role** are my "real-deal" friends who are my soul mates. They are most definitely classified as essential. These are the people who I could call at

2:00 AM requesting two hundred dollars and a shovel—and they would bring it without asking questions until afterwards. For some people, this could be a family member, a friend, or a significant other. These are the people we live and die for! These people are the ones we choose to spend time with because we genuinely want to. There is no reward for the relationship except for the fact that we truly love and appreciate their existence.

Just as we have to classify the roles for the people we choose to have in our lives—equally important, you must understand your role in other people's life. You may not be viewed as a BFF to someone that you feel close to—but you must respect the category that others put you in. We simply must understand and except the role we play in one another's life.

Be the best friend or associate that you can be in whatever aspect of the relationship you find yourself in. And this alone will make you a valuable asset to anyone affiliated with you. But attempting to force a position or status in someone else's life will cause you to be perceived as needy or clingy—and no one *who lives with purpose* wants to coddle a clingy codependent person.

True friendship is one of the most beautiful things in the world—as it transcends time, gender, race, and culture. Friendship has the transcending power to wonderfully and positively impact our lives—for it is in friendship, that we play the indispensable role of satisfying one another's needs.

What type of friends should my circle consist of?

The role of a "true friend" will look out for you when you are drinking too much at the club or party. They might suggest to you that you've had too much to drink and that you are about to make some decisions that you are going to regret tomorrow. And in another scenario, they may intervene when they see you getting yourself into a compromising situation that might endanger your life or hurt your marriage or relationship. And if there is an argument that you are involved with—they will become the voice of reason and steer you away from a confrontation. These are the kind of friends that should be found in your circle because they are the ones who hold the circle of friendship together.

What makes a friendship an interpersonal relationship?

Friendship means different things to different people depending on gender, age, and cultural background. But I personally believe the trust and loyalty proven over a period of time will automatically transfer a casual acquaintanceship to an interpersonal relationship. Throughout our lives, we will engage in an ongoing process of developing friendships.

How does the role of friendship change over time?

As we transfer from one space in life into another...leading into adulthood, our sense of self and identities shift their reference points in terms of social expectation. This simply means that as we get older that our view of life becomes more serious so that we react and respond in a more responsible manner...at least, it should. As we get older—we are expected to act more diplomatic, civil, and considerate.

More Essential roles of a relationship:

Confidants are usually your closest friend with whom you share your deepest sentiments and your darkest secrets. You turn to them for sound advice and to get their perspective on things.

Companions are friends who are always there for you through whatever you are going through. You can always count on them to stand by your side.

Collaborators are friends who usually share the same passions, interests, and ambitions. They are your "hype team," which helps you come up with ideas to propel you toward your dream and goals.

Invigorators are those friends who give you a boost of confidence and energy when you are feeling down.

They are usually the fun-seekers who will turn your frown upside down. They will keep you laughing and smiling.

Analytical Thinkers are the friends you go to for thought-provoking conversations. They challenge your intellect and are always teaching you new things. They encourage you to learn and to be interested in various topics while expanding your horizon.

Regardless of the roles people play in your life, they serve as valuable assets to you. They make the mundane exciting, and they give you hope when life seems bleak. They keep you sane when you are at your wit's end—and when you are sad, they give you a reason to laugh. Life without these essential friends would be incomplete.

Article 32

Questioning my friends?

I was having lunch on the terrace at one of my favorite restaurants in Atlanta, GA, with some friends and colleagues who were visiting me from Nashville, TN—when suddenly I heard a flamboyant voice calling out my name. When I looked to see who it was, I noticed that it was a former student of mine named David, who is openly gay. David was one of my favorite students because I had grown to respect him for the success in his life despite his life's struggles. I was glad to see him and rose from my seat to greet him. I introduced him to my friends/ colleagues, who were now standing at the table with their mouths gaped open with amazement at my acknowledgment of this obviously gay man. I offered my former student a seat at the table with my associates and me, but he declined—stating that he had business to officiate. He thanked me for the offer and flamboyantly embraced me, and said his goodbyes. My "heterosexual" friends were now relieved that this embarrassing gay man had refused the offer to sit and dine with us. They once again stared at me for an explanation, which I felt no need to give them. They had wrongly projected David's lifestyle on me by association. But, because of the awkwardness of the silence—and the opportunity to set my colleagues strait—I decided to explain the kindness I showed to my former student. I began by saying: I know you all are wondering—why is a heterosexual man like myself associated with a flamboyant homosexual? The thought was etched into their faces, so I proceeded to tell them David's story.

David is thirty-two years old and contracted the HIV virus four years ago from his now-deceased partner, who died of AIDS. It was during this time I met him as a potential student inquiring about my class. Because of the turmoil in his life with losing his lover and contracting the HIV virus, he decided to go back to school to rediscover a purpose in life—so he took my anatomy & physiology class which was part of the massage program at Georgia Medical Institute where I had taught.

David was an excellent student with a 3.9 GPA, but he suffered from depression due to the recent loss of his lover. Five months into the course, David began to miss days until he was no longer attending school. Because attrition was such a major focus at this school, the responsibility of attendance rested upon the shoulders of the instructors. So being an instructor, it was my responsibility to check on him and any other student who'd missed a series of days. I decided to go to David's house to check on him since I could no longer reach him by phone. When I arrived at David's house and knocked on the door, I noticed that the door was already ajar, so I went in and called for him. I knew something was terribly wrong…I felt it in my gut. I went through his house, calling his name,

"David, where are you?" When I found him, he was in the fetal position in the bathtub, half filled with water, whimpering, and wearing pajama bottoms. He stated to me that he had taken half of a bottle of sleeping pills with some alcohol. He said that he had attempted to end his life and was about to fulfill his demise by cutting his jugular vein until he heard my voice. That's when I notice the knife underneath his shoulder. Being lost for the right words at this crucial moment, all I could say was, *"No, you aren't!" You are not going to commit suicide or cut any blood vessels today! You have a report due in three days, and you are not going to mess up my class attrition by missing any more days!"* David looked at me, shocked as to say, *"All you can think of is your attrition?"* He began to sob loudly and then a sequence of hysterical laughs and more sobbing. I cradled him and held him like an infant for about twenty minutes. I helped him out of the tub of water and gathered the spilled pills that were scattered all over the bathroom floor. He shared how deep his pain was from the loss of his lover and how much he missed him. I felt David's deep heartache in the pit of my own stomach as he went on to say: "*I have so many seniors and clients who depend on me to keep them encouraged that the pressure and responsibility, along with my own grief—had begun to weigh me down. Mr. J.* (what my students called me), *I could no longer bare their problems compound with my own. So, thank you, Mr. J., for going outside of your duties as an instructor and being a friend.*" I sat and talked with David for a couple of hours—encouraging him and telling him how important his life was to so many people. You see…David served a senior assisted living community by offering wellness massages—so he had many senior clients depending on his services. He was their strength and their hope. After hearing David's words, all I could do was shed the tears that had already begun to fall from my eyes.

David did return back to school two days later with his report in his hand with a new zest for life. He still has bouts of depression along with emotional issues, but more than anything, David has a propelling desire not to be denied happiness. He later told me that the day I came to his house and saved his life was the day that I also saved the lives of those who were depending on him for support.

I went on to explain to my associates at the table, whose faces now quieted with embarrassment—and who were now amazed at David's influence in the community. It was at that moment that I also realized the influence that my life had on so many others. David, in return, had greatly impacted me. This experience transformed my life by restoring my sense of purpose. It has become one of my motivations for writing on the subject of finding wholeness through spirituality.

Peering into the eyes of each one of my associates at the table, I said to them: *I know some of your darkest secrets as well—just as I know David's secrets. And just as I have befriended David, a flamboyant homosexual, I have also befriended all of you. I befriended most of you at your lowest periods in life. Represented at this table where we're sitting—are Christian heterosexual men and women which I have befriended. And at this table is an abusive spouse, sex offender, one who cheats on income taxes, is unfaithful in their marriage, lies about their income, and one who doesn't pay their debts—just to mention a few of your secrets.* All the faces at the table softened with shame as I continued by saying: *that David may be an embarrassment to you because of what he displays on the outward, but he is transparent to the world. All of you, on the other hand, are impressive on the outside but have little integrity and lack real character. And you will have to bear the guilt of who you are within your own souls. So, if you care to question my friends, please start by questioning… why I am associated with you!*

If you determine a friend by the world's acceptance of them, then you have just determined that you are not a friend at all. It takes a person of confidence to stand with the unpopular.

J. Meddling

Article 33

When Intimacy Hurts

Often when we think of intimacy, we relate it to sexual intercourse, which we will address later in this article. But intimacy also relates to an emotional aspect along with the physical. Intimacy refers to *the ability to genuinely share your true self with another person and relates to the experience of closeness and connection. It is a close familiarity or friendship; or the closeness between a husband and wife*. It is clear to me that this definition of intimacy leans towards the emotional aspect.

There are some who have a fear of intimacy and will avoid getting too close or allowing others to get close to them. They might even sabotage a perfectly good relationship (intentionally or unconsciously) for fear of being hurt. I referred to this behavior as *intimacy avoidance*. This behavior is characterized by the fear of sharing close emotional or physical relationships. These same individuals may not intentionally avoid intimacy and may even long for closeness but find themselves pushing others away or sabotaging their own relationships. Many who are plagued with this kind of fear or insecurity may also wrestle with *commitment anxiety*. Those who are laden with *commitment anxiety* are typically dealing with the same fear or insecurity as those who encumber *intimacy avoidance*.

Fear of intimacy can stem from multiple reasons, including childhood abuse or neglect, unresolved emotional issues, or past hurts that have distorted their ability to trust. Overcoming the fear and anxiety can take time—both to explore and in understand the contributing factors. The first steps of healing for those who are haunted by this issue—is to allow themselves to be a little vulnerable. Open communication about one's fears or anxiety towards intimacy has to be discussed.

Categories of Intimacy Phobias:

Emotional: The inability to share your innermost feelings with another. This could be due to an early relationship experience where one shared but was judged or criticized for feeling or being a certain way. Also, people who have lost loved ones through death, divorce, imprisonment, or any other means may be left with feelings of abandonment. This trauma can prevent them from forming romantic attachments as adults as well as meaningful friendships.

Sexual: The inability to share yourself sexually. Possibly due to being told or teased about your physical body or performance. This could also reflect sexual or mental abuse where a person has been subjected to psychological trauma.

Experiential: The inability to share experiences with another because of possibly being told that you were stupid or at fault for getting yourself into a particular situation. Also, the fear of being judged morally based on past decisions.

Intellectual: The inability to share your thoughts and ideas with another. This fear or insecurity could possibly be associated with not allowing or feeling safe in being vulnerable or transparent. Perhaps you were told that your ideas or rationale is unintelligent—and you no longer feel comfortable expressing ambitions, goals, or solutions.

And all of the issues related to the category above can be factors or hindrances for anyone who has trouble with intimacy. I am certain that these four categories could include many other areas, but these are common baseline issues that many people who experience intimacy issues can relate to.

Now let's focus for a moment on a particular area relating to intimacy and vulnerability. The fear of intimacy is different from the fear of vulnerability, even though the two can be closely related. A person who is fearful of intimacy may at first be comfortable becoming vulnerable (transparent) to their trusted friends and/or family. But often, the problem begins when a person feels that those relationships are becoming too close or intimate. What typically causes the insecurity of intimacy is the fear of being abandoned when a person has allowed themselves to be vulnerable—and too much of one's self has been shared. The fear of possibly being rejected after sharing too much of one's self will usually cause the vulnerable individual to abandon or "shut down" the conversation. This "shutting down" of conversation then lead to the demise of a relationship/ friendship. The fear of abandonment is a reflection of the fear of loss—that also manifests when a person feels they have exposed too much of themselves.

Even though the fear of intimacy and vulnerability seem the same—there is, however, a major difference between the two, although they both might coexist at the same time. Nonetheless, both trigger a behavior that alternately draws a person in—then pushes them away. These fears are generally triggered by childhood experiences and manifested in adult relationships. It becomes a confusing situation for all involved when trying to determine the reason for the insecurity and pulling away if only focusing on a person's present behavior. To get to the root of a person who has intimacy fears—you must understand the initial cause of the insecurity.

Sexual Intimacy

Sexual intimacy consists of more than achieving orgasms in a relationship—but it also assists us in feeling united with another person—which brings us that overall sense of intimacy. Sex creates a bond. But there are times when one person might feel deprived of sex because of a physical or medical issue that arises with the other partner. In this case, it's nobody's fault because situations can happen that affect our sexual performances. Sometimes hormonal changes in both men and women can be a factor. But other factors (as an educational note) are vaginal dryness—which can be quite painful for women during intercourse. Other factors for women's discomfort during sex are vaginal infections, pelvic inflammatory disease (PID), vaginismus (involuntary muscle spasms of vaginal walls), or fibroids. And also, as an educational note—men who are experiencing discomfort from sex may include foreskin issues such as *Posthitis*. Posthitis is an infection of the foreskin, usually caused by fungus thriving in hot and moist conditions. Also, another male issue that can cause discomfort during intercourse is a deformity of the penis called Peyronie's or Hypospadias disease. Yet, both men and women can have allergic reactions to one another's fluids that can also cause painful intercourse. Of course, there are a host of other conditions not mentioned above, i.e., emotional issues that can interfere with the sex life—that can temporarily interfere with intimacy in a relationship. But please note that temporary issues in the bedroom should never shut down other areas of intimacy!

If either party experiences discomfort during sex, always seek medical attention—and do not try and bear through it—this is a situation that merits communication. Do not force or demand sex when your partner cannot enjoy it because of *whatever reason*—physical or emotional. Forcing sex will annihilate intimacy because intimacy is based upon love, trust, respect, and consideration.

Imposed discomforts affecting intimacy:

There are other things that can cause sexual intimacy to be hindered or broken—like imposed fetishes. The fetishes that I am speaking of are those relating to dominatrices. Even though men are thought to also be dominant—the term is implacable by definition only to women. A dominatrix is a woman who takes the dominant role in *torture-style* sex. They inflict physical pain on their partner as a part of the sexual activity. These women are referred to as practitioners of the dominatrix. Another term used for this kind of bedroom activity that men are also a part of is sadomasochism, commonly known as (S&M). Sadomasochism is the combined term referring to any person (man or woman) who likes to receive or inflict pain during sexual intercourse. And those who are a little on the conservative side in the bedroom may not particularly care for this type of bedroom energy and find it demeaning—which will also affect intimacy. Pleasing a sexually demanding partner should never cost a person their comfort or dignity.

The other element of experiencing hurt during sex relates to emotions. I hinted at this earlier under **Categories of Intimacy Phobias**. Emotional hurt can come by way of insults about one's body, comparisons to previous lovers, and criticizing one's performance...to name a few. All insults should be kept from the bedroom if a couple is focused on creating a bond and enhancing creativity in their sex life. It is very demeaning to comment negatively about your mate's body or anatomy. This kind of blatant disrespect is a real intimacy killer. Both men and women need their egos stroked during romantic engagements. Everyone wants to feel attractive and desirable to their partner. Every woman wants to feel protected and cared for by her man—and every man needs to feel respected by his woman. Both men and women alike need to know that they can be their true selves in lovemaking without the risk of mockery, judgment, or discrimination.

And finally, sex should never hurt physically or emotionally or cause one partner to feel violated, shame, remorseful, disrespected, or devalued. The acts of intimacy are one of the most bonding gifts given to humanity so let us entreat it with the honor and respect that it merits.

Article 34

Masturbation & Sex

Serving as a premarital counselor for more than six years—one of the most avoided topics was that of masturbation. This was especially true in the Christian couple's counseling sessions. Yet, masturbation is one of the most primitive and private practice activities among people of all races, creeds, colors, and even religions. It is interesting to me how some people (usually religious people) view masturbation as being the "great dark evil," and yet I am discovering through statistics and surveys that I have personally done—that religious folks are some of the biggest practitioners of the act. This may be due to the fact that in most religious communities—sex before marriage is prohibited. And the only other solution for relieving one's self of sexual tension is through the private act of masturbation. In my years of doing couple's counseling—I noticed people evading the topic seeing that religious folks generally viewed masturbation as being a leud act—and therefore were uncomfortable talking about it.

Masturbation is defined: As self-excitement or stimulation of the genitalia. It is also called *onanism* in the biblical texts—meaning coitus interruptus and in some studies as "self-abuse." The denotation that masturbation is self-abuse, therefore making it a sin—

is restricted only to a few religious interpretations. The term "coitus interruptus" translated is the "interruption" of sexual intercourse—specifically with the purpose of withdrawing the penis from the vagina before ejaculation. It is also more commonly known as the "withdrawal method," in preventing pregnancy. In the biblical texts where it is named after "Onan," a man mentioned in the Old Testament in Genesis 38: 9-10 who ejaculated onto the ground to keep from impregnating his deceased brother's wife. This was considered a sin that Onan committed because it was a selfish act that went against the customs and the Mosaic law. Onan broke the law of tradition by not impregnating his deceased brother's wife, which was the custom of that day to ensure that the family name of the deceased brother would continue on by the sons of Onan's seed. You would have to reference Genesis 38: 9-10 to understand the customs of that time and the reason why it was considered a sin. Nevertheless, masturbation is a reality in most cultures and is not an act of sin or viewed as self-abuse as mentioned earlier.

In gathering information for this book, I have talked to many people about their view on the matter— and had them to commit to doing surveys on this subject. I would like to share with you what I thought as interesting comments that my surveyors made when I ask the general question of *Why do you do it?* Of course, the obvious answers from both men and women were that *masturbation is simply pleasurable*!

But I heard a few interesting responses that caught my attention. One woman stated to me that when she masturbates, she feels a deep sense of connection with herself. She went on to say that after masturbating—it was like falling in love with herself. I then asked her to explain, and she said: *"When I masturbate, I feel a connection with myself just as I would feel that connection with a lover. I feel a sense of respect and self-appreciation in knowing that I do not have to sleep around to experience sexual fulfillment—I am self-contained."* She continued by saying that masturbation was emotionally safer for her because she did not have to contend with the possibility of later being dumped after giving up sex. The women who took my survey generally stated that masturbation freed them from the worry of getting STDs or getting pregnant. Other women added that orgasms from masturbation were more intense than that from penetration.

These statements engaged me into a processing of theories and ideals as to why some people (particularly women) feel more enjoyment in the act of masturbation than sexual intercourse. When I asked a group of 200 men about masturbation, a good 97% of them felt that it was as natural as breathing. Most of the men stated that they find it to be an enjoyable act even after having sex with their mates—and that it was simply a casual entertainment. Both men and women expressed that after having their first or second child, that masturbating was their favorite pastime. This probably lends to the busy schedules that come with having a family. The energy levels of both partners in a family setting—are typically much lower than that of singles, or couples who have no children. And when the children come alone—usually one partner feels *attention deprived*. Typically, it is the man who experiences this deprivation. However, some women expressed feeling neglected by their men after child/ children came into the picture. When I communicated to the men about their women feeling neglected after having a child—they concurred that their lack of attentiveness was due to exhaustion. The business of taking care of a wife and kids not only fatigued them physically but emotionally as well. The guys went on to express that they had to incorporate more working hours to support their growing families. Their energy levels had waned as a result of the new demands that was on them.

Having children in the home can temporarily cripple the couple's intimacy at some point. But that is a very natural occurrence, especially when the children become the main focus of the family. It is, therefore, crucial to the well-being of a relationship for couples to find time to romance one another during this period. It is not healthy for the relationship to negate one another's needs because of children. Both men and women have the same basic needs in a relationship— the need for love, respect, assurance, devotion, and pleasure. With that being said, my group of

227

interviewees and surveyors said that masturbation was of great importance—especially in the family dynamics involving having small children.

For many, masturbation provides a series of benefits, such as: releasing sexual tension, aiding in better sleeping, reducing stress, relieving menstrual cramps and muscle tension, and strengthening muscle tone in the pelvic and anal area. Masturbation can even play a role in helping with erectile dysfunction (ED) in that it can help relieve anxiety and any other psychological issues related to ED. Being able to get an erection during masturbation may cause a man to feel more confident about himself when needing to maintain an erection with his partner. And if there is guilt associated with masturbation—getting an understanding of why you're experiencing the "guilt" need to be evaluated and understood. If we as human beings feed, bathe and clothe ourselves—shouldn't it seem natural that we would also take care of our own sexual need by pleasuring ourselves? Too many of us have adopted unmerited convictions that have been passed down through religious belief systems. Let us stop judging and convicting ourselves over self-acts that are exclusively our choice in the confines of our privacy.

Article 35

Understanding *"Self"* in Sexuality *(View on Men)*

Sexuality is defined as the *capacity for sexual feelings or the quality of being sexual*. In my expressed laymen's terms—sexuality is simply one's view or perception of how a person sees or feels about themselves sexually. Men's and women's sexuality can be affected by many factors, including culture, upbringing, individual personality, and a *sense of self*. When speaking of a *sense of self*—I am relating to the ego factor, which lends to how a man views himself as it corresponds to his sexual needs and or performances. The ego is that sense of self-importance that often exalts itself over others. Please understand that having an ego isn't necessarily a bad thing when we understand its connection with self-preservation. With that being said…there is nothing wrong when a person (male or female) is being aware of their own need and desires, as I mentioned in Article 12 **Why Should I Be Selfish**. Though we are taught that to be selfish or self-centered is a negative thing, it is simply the act of being self-aware. Now let's look at how all of this tie into male sexuality.

If a man has been sexually abused as a child, ridiculed or mocked by former lovers about his sexual performance, or teased about the size of his genitalia...he will potentially create an unhealthy view of himself. This can cause him to have serious struggles with his sexuality because his self-esteem has been bruised. Sometimes it can be the self-infliction of a man's perception about his height, weight, or education that can inflict the greatest harm to his sexuality. Though men are usually more assertive when it comes to sex—these insecurities about themselves can inhibit them from projecting confidence when it involves the approach to sexual situations. Some of these inhibitions are generated from sexual, physical, or verbal abuses that he may have suffered from youth. If a man has been abused in any one of these areas as a child, his lack of self-confidence might manifest in a relationship as brutishness. He may feel the need to display dominance and power in his adult relationships to compensate for his inabilities and lack of power as a child. He may also lack sensitivity towards his partners in intimacy because of these past issues. If living with guilt, anger, frustration, or any ill feelings—has become his mode of survival—his ability to be an effective communicator with a partner will also become problematic. Abuses in one's life can wreak havoc on a person's ability to communicate his or her feelings if they feel inadequate within themselves.

Verbal abuse on a child often leaves more permanent scars in the psyche than physical abuse because of the self-identity issues that usually remain.

What I've seen when humans are broken or damaged in their psyche is a profound need to feel *whole*, complete, and accepted. Whether male or female, we all have the same basic need—the need to feel accepted.

Men, just like women, need to feel attractive and accepted in order to be balanced in their sexuality. A man flirting is a healthy sign that he is in a good emotional *place* and possesses a healthy image of *self*. Another ego or self-esteem boost that I have observed with men is when they become fathers. For some men, having a baby gives them a sense of manhood which makes them feel more potent and sexier. Yes, men feel sexy, too—just like women! And like women, men should celebrate themselves when something grand has been accomplished. This form of showing self-appreciation adds to his healthy emotional state—which consequently boosts his *image of self*. It is not about him being macho or egotistic—but about honoring himself and giving attention to his own emotional needs. And when our emotional needs are fulfilled—we feel good about ourselves and our sexuality. And as we embrace our sexuality as men—let us be mindful to think well of ourselves and to live in the bliss and sexual excitement we were created in.

Article 36

Understanding *"Self"* in Sexuality
(View on Women)

It is from a woman's *sense of self* that her sexuality or interest in sex is formed. Sexuality is the quality or state of being sexual. In my words: *sexuality is one's view or perception of how they see or feel about themselves sexually.* Many women (at least in my observation) are challenged in matters of their sexuality. I am not speaking of challenges in the sense of sexual orientation as it relates to lesbianism. But I am speaking of the challenges that women have in seeing themselves as sexy—those who lack sexual confidence because of their obscured *sense of self.* I have personally observed that Western-cultured women are more sexually inhibited in comparison to women in other major countries. I am not suggesting that this is inclusive to ALL Western-cultured women, but my personal observation is that women in European countries are much more liberal and expressive about their sexual needs and preferences than Western women. I have also observed more sexual liberties in other parts of the world in comparison to America. But my admonishment to women is to possess and maintain a healthy perception of their sexuality by doing things for themselves that make them feel beautiful and loved. I encourage women to treat themselves to simple pleasantries like a day at the spa or the hair salon. Having a manicure and pedicure, or buying a new pair of shoes—may be all that's needed to change your perception of *self*.

Women who have a poor sexual image of themselves will often experience unfulfilled sexual relationships. Sometimes a poor sexual image of one's self is rooted in sexual abuse, physical abuse, or emotional/ verbal abuse.

Because women are typically more emotionally based, verbal communication plays a huge role in a woman's psyche when it comes to her *feeling sexual*. In order for her to have a healthy sexual relationship, she must be free to communicate any insecurity she might have about sex or about herself—without feeling judged. Securing a woman's image of herself is the doorway to her being able to feel good about who she is as a sexual being. So, the need for compliments from others, and even from herself by means of self-validation—is something women thrive on. And as a partner, allowing a woman to have an open dialogue about her fears and expectations is the foundation for a healthy sexual relationship. For women who aren't as sexually liberated—an understanding of their sexuality is essential before they can experience true ecstasy in lovemaking. For many women, ecstasy does not happen automatically when there are insecurities. If a woman is to experience sexual fulfillment from her partner on an emotional/ spiritual level—she must feel validated. This validation can come from herself by way of positive self-talk, from her partner or even from her friends who reminds her of how beautiful and smart she is. Validation also helps her in possessing that sense of sexual confidence that also stems from being admired and appreciated by her mate. And for some women who aren't as sexually confident as others—it will takes some practice and self-observation to master the sexual fluidity and confidence that comes with being sexy.

Women who are shy or inexpressive in the bedroom are often dealing with identity issues about their sexuality. Once again, this is not an all-inclusive fact because some women just aren't verbally expressive in bed. However, in my personal observation of surveys that I took—African American women in the US had a higher rate of sexual inhibitions than other groups of women in the US. In a multicultural discussion group with only women, the African American women—more than all others, posed and shared their innermost insecurity relating to sex. I personally believe that these issues take their roots all the way back to slavery when Africans were stripped of their identity, culture, beliefs, and pride. African women were separated from their husbands and children and were made to be the *slaver's* sex slaves, along with many other degrading duties. These women were simply raped physically and emotionally—losing all sense of self-value. It is my humble opinion—that this tragedy could have played a role into the psyche of black women—who inherited their African ancestors' sense of degradation. This kind of subjection, in my opinion, distorted black women's identity of self and has been passed down for generations. (Read this book as a reference to sexual history and women in slavery: Horny & Saved by Sandra L. Snowden, pages 16-17, Historical Evolution of Sex). Another factor for the loss of sexual identity among black women (and women in general) may be related to what has been taught in churches and synagogues. The teachings of submission and subjection, the suppression of sexual feelings alone with generations of inherited degradations—may be partly responsible for the sexual insecurities that many women in our culture have. For this reason, women of every background, creed, and ethnicity struggle at some point in their life—with the issues of their sexuality.

In some countries, social conditioning dictates that sexual pleasure is only for the man and that women are only to be the providers of pleasure and children and not the recipient. Even where this ideology is not verbally taught, it is however—culturally prominent and expected. This mindset gives some understanding as to why these musical videos show multiple women half-naked dancing seductively around one man—or men slapping women on their behinds with a dog chain around the women's necks. The perception of women being in servitude to men is alive and well in many cultures—though servitude can be displayed in many other ways other than the one I've mentioned. This perception of women being subservient to men is fed subliminally into the mind of our society by way of media every day.

Women who have not awakened to their *feminine divinity* have adopted the mentality of worthlessness. Their *sense of self* is distorted by how the culture views them and treats them as invaluable objects. No wonder women are losing their sense of sexiness towards guys while some have turned to other women sexually because of feeling devalued by men. A woman will not have a good sense of her sexuality when she is unable to see her value.

This is why it is important for a woman to give value to herself. She should make the time to pamper herself—not wait for someone else to show her the love that she already has for herself. This self-romance allows her to grow more in love with herself—becoming more confident in her expressions and sexuality. Self-romancing is simply doing those things for yourself that make you, as a woman, feel sexy, loved, and respected. To add to the suggestions that I made earlier about women treating themselves—include to that list—occasionally send roses to yourself, buy sexy lingerie, treat yourself to a meal at a fine dining restaurant, or plan a picnic with yourself. Doing these activities alone may initially feel a little awkward at first—or you might find yourself feeling embarrassed about picnicking by yourself—but these simple activities give a huge boost to the self-image and lend to self-love. Showing this kind of attention to yourself will help to validate your love for *yourself* and will strengthen your sense of sexuality.

Article 37

Breaking Influences

Some of the most difficult influences to break are those imposed upon us as children. These same influences or habits can become the most dominant controlling factors in our adult lives. An "influence" can be understood as anything, person, or situation that sways or causes us to lean towards an opinion—creating our belief system.

Sometimes people are unwillingly swayed to the belief system of another in order to get along with them and to maintain peace. This is especially true if they are living together under the same roof. Often the need to maintain commonality (the need to fit in) is another reason people settle into other's beliefs. No matter the reason, we are all influenced at some time or another into idealism or belief systems that do not match our core convictions. Most of us believe the things we're taught growing up as being *true*, but often those things do not connect with our authentic convictions. This is the reason why some become dissuaded into belief systems that were not taught to them as children. But our authentic convictions or *inner self,* which I recognize as the God aspect of our *being*, knows all truth and will not agree with that which is false. Even if you are unable to rationalize why something you've been told is wrong—your *inner self* knows the truth—

even if you can't verbalize it. Often, people will have conflicting feelings about the things they grew up believing. But if they are unable to disprove those things because of the lack of enlightenment—they might find themselves governed by conflicting beliefs. This is to say, that they will have trepidation or doubts about what they've learned as being factual. The conflict was there all alone while holding onto a *perceived* truth that could not yet be understood or recognized.

Having the right influences in our life is vital because it is through influence that we learn and understand behavior appropriateness and separate truths from facts. This is to say that the people we hold dear to us have the ability to mold our perception of the world around us. However, it is necessary to break the influences that take us outside of our core convictions—which are the things we believe in our heart. Any influence that prevents us from adhering to our own personal convictions should be shunned observed closely using our critical thinking skills. If our core convictions become intertwined with misguided information through years of wrong teachings and bad influences—it becomes the job of our *inner self* to bring us enlightenment. We can grow up believing that what we were taught (about any given thing) as being true can turn out to be misinformation. And this is why we must live by our own constitution of right and wrong as long as it does not harm another.

We can only live by the enlightenment that we have at any given period of our life. This is to say that as children, we must believe what adults teach us because we have not yet lived or experienced life to know what's true. But once we live and have our own life experiences, we must break away or either re-evaluate what it is that we actually believe—and why we believe what we believe. This is where a maturing and enlightened individual applies critical thinking skills.

Perhaps, if we are totally off-based in our belief system, I believe it becomes the job of the Universe/God to teach us through life experiences what is truth. No one has the infinite wisdom to teach or lead us on the path that is meant for our *individual* lives except God. If another tries to teach or lead us contrary to our own convictions, we will usually end up emotionally marred if we surrender to their belief. When people become marred by bad influences or teachings and lose sight of their own core convictions, the bad influences have to be broken in order for them to become whole. When our perception of *self* becomes devalued by bad influences and misinformation—wrong decisions for our life always follow. An example of this is when a child grows up being told that they will never amount to anything—and they fulfill that imposed prophecy to living a life of destruction. This is an example of bad influences and misinformation devastating someone's life.

Negative influences are not easily broken because they are often intertwined into the core of our convictions—which are often rooted in years of misguided beliefs. Therefore, we must do diligent in breaking these influences by changing our association. If misguided beliefs are a result of what we've been told as a child, then new positive influences will have to take place. I stated in the beginning that the hardest influences to break are those imposed upon us as children. I believe the best way to reprogram "old mindsets" is by finding new associations. When you transition away from people of negative influence, do not bother trying to explain your reasons for transitioning away from them—for they will never understand your rationalization until they become enlightened on their own path to enlightenment.

Look for people who are living in the "consciousness" that you are seeking. Associate with those who see you in a way in which you want to be seen—those who perceive you to be a good person. Observe those who live by their own convictions. These individuals may not be the most popular in mainstream circles. So, prepare yourself to be among those who may not live by the orders of popular opinions. Seekers of truth usually run in smaller groups. These are the people (in my opinion) who are on the spiritual path looking for universal harmony and not possessing a hidden religious agenda. Seekers of truth are usually searching for their own way to wholeness and are not interested in converting others into their belief. Seekers of truth understand that every person has a built-in roadmap that can only be followed by the one who possesses it. They also understand that the "truth" for someone else's life might be different from their own. Anyone who is trying to convert another to their belief system by stating that they have the "One Truth," avoid them! The Universe is multifaceted and carries many truths.

Secondly, to break negative influences—a change in our perception of who we are has to be re-introduced *to* and *through* our own thought process. We must stop agreeing with the negative situations in our lives and claiming them as our reality. Stop feeding into the negative belief systems that things must always be burdensome in life. If we are not making the money that we want to make, stop saying, "I'm broke." If we are feeling lonely, stop confessing to loneliness. If you are overweight, underweight, unemployed, fearful, sickly, or anything that creates negative feelings—stop proclaiming it as a part of your reality. Instead, start saying to *yourself* that my income is abundant, I am not lonely but surrounded by many friends, my weight is healthy, I am not fearful but courageous, and I am not sickly but live in perfect health. In order for the outside situations to change, the inside perception must change first. Having a paradigm shift of *self* is essential for external transformation.

We cannot change other people's lives by simply wanting them to change. Our responsibility to ourselves is to secure our own *wholeness* by breaking the negative influences that hinder our healthy perception of *self*. We are the beauty that we believe ourselves to be!

We change our lives when we change our association—we change the world when the world sees us changed.

J. Meddling

Article 38

The Potency of Touch

Human beings can survive fairly normally without sight, smell, taste, and hearing, but not without the ability to touch or feel. Out of our "five senses," touch scientifically is proven to be the most vital of them all. When we understand that there are approximately ten thousand nerve sensors in one square inch of skin, we can then appreciate the intricately designed sensory of touch. But this type of touch sensory is not the primary target of this subject matter that I am speaking of. I will address the power of physical touch—but the ability to touch the human spirit through words and deeds, is the direction of my focus. But both aspects of touch are powerful tools that we all carry in our toolbelts. Touch transcends the physical into the spiritual arena—and we cannot survive or maintain emotional balance without it—because touch is associated with connecting with another person's spirit.

In the late 1960s, in a German hospital in the maternity ward where they kept a group of premature newborns—a female housekeeper would come by every night to pick up the trash from the nursery area. She had made a nightly habit of touching and holding the six premature infants that were closest to the doorway where all the trash was gathered. This was done over a period of three weeks. An observation was made that the six premature babies that the housekeeper touched on a daily basis were out growing the other preemies in leaps and bounds. The doctors ran tests and checked their records for feeding schedules in trying to understand the reasoning behind this obvious growth. The doctors could not find any variance in the care given to the six infants—until the housekeeper was later discovered giving the six infants *that* extra attention. So, the doctors concluded that it was, without a doubt, because of the physical attention that these six babies were receiving from the housekeeper—was responsible for their exponential growth.

Touch is powerful and crucial to human survival—for it is in the touch that an infusion of life and vitality is imparted from one to another. In ancient times before modern medicine (as we know it), people would be physically healed by the simple laying on of hands. Evil energies, or demons as commonly related to—was forced out of people by a touch from those who possessed supernatural good energies. Whether we believe in the healing gifts by the laying on of hands or not, the principle of touch causes a physiological change—yet holds scientific truth

Having taught anatomy, physiology, and pathology—one thing that I know from a physiological aspect is that when you injure any part of your body and bring your hands to the injured area for comfort, a super influx of blood rushes to the area. This response is called hyperemia—which is the process of oxygen filled blood suppling an organ or other parts of the body. Blood is naturally flowing throughout the body at all times—but it is scientifically proven that twenty percent more blood flows to the area when a physical touch aids the injury. I believe this to be the reason why we instinctively grab or hold an area when we feel pain in it.

There is another form of touch that is not physical, which I mentioned at the beginning of this article. This form of touch is directed to the spirit of a person. Dr. Wayne Dyer stated in his audiobook (Power of Intention) that one of the ways in which we declare the power found in non-physical touch is when we offer a public act of kindness. How we treat and interact with our fellow man promotes a physiological change in both our own bodies as well as the bodies of the observers. When an act of kindness is done publicly, serotonin is released into the nervous system, causing a warm, harmonious sensation in all who witness the act. Serotonin is a hormone that acts as a neurotransmitter providing a sensation of happiness and well-being. It is the "feel-good drug" that our bodies naturally make when a good deed is done. Even the one committing the act of goodness is benefited.

I also believe that touch encompasses the effect that words have on our physiology. We use terms such as "I was touched by their story" or "she really touched my heart." This is proof that our body has stimuli to verbalization. We as humans need validation—which is transferred through touch, and allows us to experience a sense of empowerment and wholeness. This is why (as human beings)—we need acknowledgement when we do a great job at work. They appreciation that we show to one another is felt on a deep spiritual level. This type of recognition not only gives validation to one's worth—but it also boosts morale while warming the human heart. It is the simple complements and considerations that lay the groundwork for healing within a person on every level. The body, mind, and spirit are all positively impacted.

Have you ever been told that an outfit you were wearing was really nice—or that you were very pretty or handsome? How did that make you feel? Did you blush a little? It probably made you feel warm and appreciated causing you to blush. That blushing was the physiological change that took place in your body without anyone physically touching you. Blood rushes to the capillaries of your skin, causing peach color pigmentation. This shows how much power our words possess and the changes it causes on a spiritual level. If we as human beings can have this much of a positive impact on one another, why don't we offer more of this healthy "touch" in a world starving for love and recognition?

Nothing can touch the human heart as deeply as words—so choose your words with care.

J. Meddling

Article 39

The Psychology of Dieting

People have become obsessed with losing weight and getting slim. There is such an insatiable need for looking attractive and being fit in our society—that new diet products are popping up everywhere and nearly every day. Dieting products and surgeries for weight reduction have become a multi-million-dollar industry. After spending hundreds and even thousands of dollars on weight loss, some will unfortunately—continue struggling with weight issues or eating disorders. This is because many do not understand the dynamic role that the psyche plays in dieting. The human mind, I believe—is the most powerful factor in losing, gaining, or maintaining weight. How we think and perceive can have a physiological effect on our metabolism.

Several years ago, I taught anatomy, physiology, and pathology as a part of a massage therapy course at Georgia Medical Institute. In addition to teaching massage modalities and ethics, I would encourage my students to eat and live healthily as therapists. I told them that the best diet to be on is the diet that allows you to eat "moderately" everything you want to eat. I stressed to them that focusing on what you cannot have—only create more desire for the food that you believe you shouldn't have. When we determine that something is "bad" for us—it actually manifests a negative response in our body if we participate in that *thing*. It is amazing how powerful our mind and thoughts can become when we focus on something. So, if you believe that a particular food is bad for you—it can create a negative response in your body—even if it really wasn't. This concept is applicable to anything you give negative or positive energy to. Your body will adapt to whatever you bombard your mind to believe. Science has proven this repeatedly! You become (for all intent and purpose) what you proclaim.

I continued by telling my students that if they would only incorporate a few simple exercises in their daily routine (which I incorporated into my classes each morning for thirty minutes)—that they would begin to lose weight with only minimum effort. I reminded the students every day for thirty days that *they would become what they proclaimed* themselves to be. And in those thirty days—the students who were interested in weight loss began to lose weight on a consistent basis. They simply put their belief into action (by way of exercise), and this action manifested what they desired.

In an article written by Holly Pinafore, "How Your Thoughts Affect Your Metabolism,"—Marc David, M.A., nutritionist and psychologist who founded the Psychology of Eating Institute in Colorado, shares common thoughts on the subject. Marc David M.A. explains that 80% of digestion, relaxation, assimilation, and calorie-burning power come from CPDR- cephalic phase digestive response. Cephalic means (of the head)—and studies showed that we needed to experience more than full bellies when trying to diet. We also need to experience taste, aroma, and satisfaction in order to increase our digestion and calorie-burning capacities which derive from "thought." Marc continues by saying if I can paraphrase, that when we shovel our food down in a rush or guilty manner (believing a particular food to be bad), we cannot properly digest or enjoy the taste of the food. When we stress over what is safe to eat, our bodies go into a defense mode, causing hydrocortisone (cortisol) and insulin to release. This steroid hormone (cortisol) is secreted by the adrenal cortex and acts on carbohydrate metabolism and stores in the fatty tissues, causing weight gain.

So, we can see how our thoughts can make a huge impact on our weight when we choose to *dread* certain foods instead of simply enjoying them. This fear of food only increases the stress hormones cortisol and insulin.

Helping my students to simply change their mindset about "bad foods" propelled them into healthier lifestyles and optimum health. And the stretching and flexing exercises that my students incorporated were so effortless that they would incorporate these simple techniques in their homes after school or work. Many of them, to this very day, continue to lose weight or maintain their size as a result of the exercises I taught them. One of my students in particular—was grossly overweight when she began my course. She was someone with extremely poor dieting habits. But this student continued with the new mindset about food and continued her exercises two years after finishing my course. When I saw her two, and half years later, I did not recognize her. It was only after staring into the student's face that I remembered who she was. She carried herself with such confidence—something she did not possess years earlier when she first came to my class. I remembered how she used to struggle with self-esteem and weight issues—but not anymore! Needless to say, how excited I was to see a life so drastically but wonderfully changed because of the knowledge that I had imparted about the psychology of dieting.

What we must understand is that when we believe a certain food to be an enemy to our health—we will manifest that false-hood into our reality. To further stress my point from a biblical perspective, this not only applies to food but anything that we have strong emotions or convictions about. In the Holy Bible, Romans 14:14 speaks to dietary issues and reads: *...but to him who thinks anything to be unclean, to him it is unclean.*

Discarding negative beliefs about foods would be a good place to start in the process of getting healthy. It would be a good idea to remove the word "diet" from our health vocabulary. The word "diet" currently carries a negative connotation or energy—losing its true meaning, which is "A Way of Life." The way we eat should become an everyday practice and not just a regiment to lose or gain weight. Another thing to consider for maintaining a healthy mindset about food is to eat your food in the present. When we eat in the present—we focus our attention on the flavor and presentation of the food—we observe the colors and aroma. We should look forward to our meal and savor the experience of eating. Anticipating our meals before actually eating causes our mouth to salivate—creating saliva, which is the first neutralizing chemical process of breaking food down and preparing it for the stomach. Simply taking the time to chew your food into a liquid state before swallowing—allows two enzymes called *amylase* and *lingual lipase* to mix with your food. *Amylase* and *lingual lipase* are enzymes that breaks down starches and fats. These natural chemicals prepare the food for the stomach—so that the stomach doesn't work as hard to bread down foods. This alone will aid in maintaining a healthy stomach and colon.

I personally believe that having and showing gratitude for our provision by giving thanks—places us into a healthier mindset. These simple suggestions will cause a healthy physiological change to take place in the body as well. These are the things I told my students years ago—and is a part of what I believe and practice today. Eat everything you want—but in moderation. Love your life and get plenty of exercises—and your body and life will always treat you well!

Article 40

Misinterpreting Human Behavior

Often, we judge people's characters by their actions, and we ultimately categorize people as being bad or good based on that observation. But I am of the opinion that behavior and deeds do not adequately reflect what is in the heart of the individual. How a person sees themselves in their own minds really defines who they are—even if their behavior contradicts the perception of how they view themselves. It is our hearts/ perception of ourselves that defines the truth of who we are. The Bible states: (paraphrased) "*that human beings judge the outward appearance, but only God knows the heart of man.*" (1 Samuel 16:7). Religious people will counter that statement by quoting (Matthew 7:16) that read: "*You shall know them by their fruits...*," insinuating that people are what they do—or that people are known by their actions or behavior. But people need time to mature into the masterpiece that they are innately. And what I'm referring to when I say innately—I am talking about living like the essence of God within them. Many of the people that we wrongly judge or characterize as "bad" are still in the *seed* stage of their life. Most of us cannot identify a mustard seed from its full-grown tree. Thus, many people are still in that seed—where behavior and intentions are often misinterpreted. Even when the "tree" is yet reaching maturity, there can be confusion about what type of tree it is unless you know the seed that was planted. And unless you are a carpologist (one who studies fruits and seeds), you will not be able to recognize or identify a seed if you saw it. The carpologist represents a mature, discerning individual who understands that people need time to germinate, blossom and grow. And in this context—the one who understands spiritual development.

People go through many seasons in their lives, and in the winter months, just like trees, we cannot tell one tree from another when the leaves and fruit of that tree have fallen off. The same is true when people are in the winter transition of their lives. How many of us have gotten drunk in our lives? We may have acted in an embarrassing manner but does that single act constitute us as an alcoholic? Have any of us ever experimented with drugs? If yes, does that certify you as a drug addict? How many people, out of curiosity, have had a sexual encounter with someone of the same gender? Does that automatically make them homosexual if they were going through an experimental phase in their life? We could continue this list of questioning—but I am certain you get the gist of my point.

So not understanding what stage of life a person is in (at any given time) can lead us to judge them wrongly when we see behaviors that we deemed inappropriate. The Apostle Paul states in Romans 7: 18- 23 (paraphrased), "...*the good that I want to do, I*

don't do, but rather I end up doing the opposite—the
bad that I do not want to do, that's what I end up doing.
Whenever I want to do good, the evil that I do not want
to do—has a way of taking over. I have come to the
conclusion that there is nothing inherently good in this
flesh because it's always fighting against the real me
who is a righteous and spiritual being."

God's nature or *seed of truth* within us is constantly manifesting its way into our conscious levels. But the growth may not look like what many might consider as growth—but might appear as inappropriate behavior. How many of us have been caught in a bad situation where our reputation was on the line—but later, that experience changed the trajectory of our life for the good? This is simply the way life is when we are growing through our life experiences. Our experiences in life are grooming us into what we are to become. We are not a finished work until we become more like our Creator—so this is a life-long process that continues until we reach the grave. But our growth will be recognized alone the way. Our growth mirrors the process of a baby's birth into this world. Physically, a birth is not a "pretty" sight—but it takes that agonizing, bloody, and painful experience in order for that life to come into this world. It is absolutely no different in spiritual conception. God gives birth within us—and in time, we mature into a whole *being*. God's seed is already in us, which makes us innately good—but

257

during the growth process—this reality might be unrecognizable.

Make no mistake about it—I am not condoning irresponsible and careless living. My purpose is to encourage those who have been wounded by the misjudgments of others—and who may be feeling that they are good for nothing because of the mistakes that they have made. I am not defending those who take pleasure in doing harm to others—but am addressing those who are having hiccups in their life. In fact, I believe that the difference between people who are *purposefully* a menace to society—is that on a subconscious level, manifesting who they *really* are on the inside. The one who relishes imposing fear, dominance, hatred and any other ill-behavior—I would consider as evil or misguided. This is contrary to those I've been making references to throughout this article. Because, anyone who feels bad about their disruptive behaviors on a subconscious level will eventually turn from those actions. The person who feels remorseful or shame for the inappropriateness that they do—I would consider as an indication that this person is unconsciously reaching for their wholeness.

What a person enjoys is the expression of their true nature. But if a person feels guilty about the acts they are committing—it is not reflective of that person's true character. The true essence of every "good" individual is to be at peace and harmony with themselves. Therefore, if you are unhappy with yourself and are feeling conviction about any aspect of your life—you are not yet experiencing the wholeness of your true essence.

The man who finds peace within himself—has found peace with God.

J. Meddling

Article 41

Loosing *Self* in Religious Addictions

In the seventeen years of serving as a counselor and life coach—I have learned that many are conflicted with being their authentic self for fear of offending the expectations of their religion. This conflict exists because religion, by design, is meant to confine, restrict and constrain *perceived* inappropriate human behavior. Yet, we all have our personal opinions and beliefs about what we believe to be appropriate and inappropriate. I believe that God never meant for humans to live under the restrictions that some religious authoritarians require us to live by. I believe that many of the restrictions that religion has placed upon people are not exactly the order of God but of men to control the activities of its citizens. However, I do believe in societal order—but this order need only be enforced upon those who step out of its protection.

Order is indeed protection for its citizens, but it should never dictate a person's freedom to be or express who they are as long as their expression does not cause harm to others. Restricting a person from being who they are is a violation of our humanity. We are spiritual beings learning how to exist in the confinement of human form. We innately resist anything that does not correspond with the identity of our essence, which is *free spiritedness*. I am not suggesting that there should not be structure and laws binding to ordinances. However, when *religious laws* dictate the private activities of adult individuals—this is where I believe the conflict begins. I bear my own prejudice and biases against what I personally consider immoral activities, but I understand that the activities of others do not have to be a part of my experience. I simply believe that everyone has the right to choose what's appropriate and inappropriate for them, whether I or anyone else agrees. And if these inappropriate behaviors step outside of the guidelines of what the law of our land says, then repercussions must be initiated.

We are born into this human existence with the understanding that rules and regulations are in place. Therefore, we by our very existence in this era—and in this human form except these ordinances. And as citizens, we have the right to guard against *religious expectations*—that's imposed upon us by society. As long as we abide by the laws that govern us as citizens—we are required to follow the expectations of religious communities. I humbly believe that our focus should be on the things that we desire for our lives—while allowing others the freedom to create their own experiences. We do not have to bash or be angry toward those who do not favor our belief system.

Religion is not a constitution of God but a man-made ordinance that is supposed to be established upon divine truths established by God. But the question is, "Who really knows what is in the mind of God?" Who is qualified, or to whom or what—have we trusted to be the *absolute* mouthpiece of the All-Knowing? Religion can only imply God's expressed *will*. And I know many of the readers are probably thinking that we have holy books and manuscripts indicating God's laws or sentiments. And I would 100% agree with you on that point. I have personally been a student of the bible for more than forty years—and have adeptly studied from many other holy books and texts. I have studied from the Dead Sea Scrolls (English translation), the Quran, The Ethiopian Orthodox Bible (that includes the missing books of the bible and considered the second oldest bible in the world). I have also studied from the Bhagavad Gita (holy book of the Hindus), The teachings of Buddhism and many others. And the conclusion that I have arrived at is that all of these books were written centuries ago and have gone through multiple translations. And they were written by people who did not really understand how and why things occurred. So, they attributed phenomena's—such as droughts, famines, tornados, astrological events, plagues and etc.—to deities that they assumed was angry with mankind. The people of those days were inundated by the moral values of the era in which they lived. And even then—the laws were not inclusive to all but showed biasness towards certain individuals. One example of this is when they advocated stoning for adulterous wives—but no sanctions for an adulterous husbands or man. And the list of moral values to which these writers ascribed (that would be repugnant in this era), is nearly endless. So, as I have referenced many time throughout this book—I do not have full confidence in any of the holy books. But I will add that in these holy books are enough basic, common sense, moral concepts—for anyone who wants to be a decent human—to live by. And even though I am an avid reader and student of most of the "holy texts"—for me to except ANY of them as the unadulterated word of God is still a challenge for me.

Some religions teach that we are not free unless we live by certain guidelines from a particular holy book or reference. Religion does not teach us to be critical thinkers but rather dictates how we should think. The problem I see with most religions is that it does more dictating and controlling rather than teaching us how to observe the constantly changing world around us. Many people see religion as the angry taskmaster— who is to be feared and not questioned. This is why there are so many "holy wars" going on in the world— people attempting to control others based on their religious beliefs. If everyone believes that their cause/ belief is the right one (the one ordained by God)—and attempt to impose that belief on others—it will only keep the world in disharmony. If everyone understood their God-given power (which embodies each one of us), there would be no need to rule, control, or constrain the practices of others. There would be no need to compete for sovereignty—for we would only draw those who are in harmony with us—leaving the unharmonious or *unbelieving* out of our realities. This is to simply suggest that we only have these wars because our focus is on those who oppose rather than placing our interest and energy in seeking out those who are in harmony with what we believe. The world is encompassing enough for every religious belief—without any of us clashing in belief systems if we'd change our intentions and focus.

Religion demands attention to the ordinances given to rituals such as going to church, not fornicating, not killing or stealing, taking the Lord's Supper or Eucharist, fasting, and observing Holy Days—to name a few. It is based on doing "deeds" that do not add to one's closeness to God. There is nothing wrong with any of these observances, in my opinion, but when one seeks to understand the *essence of the inner self* or the God within—the pure focus is sometimes lost by the sentiments of doing good deeds to gain enlightenment. In other words, people try and find God (who is already within them) by doing religious acts. But the essence of who we are (which is God) is being subdued by the very acts that are supposed to give awareness of who God is. We seek to obtain *Godliness* through acts and good deeds when *Godliness* is already within us.

Even our personal aspirations get cloudy with religious dogma. For example, A person aspires to be a multi-millionaire, but their religious teachings instruct them that all monies made beyond taking care of the basic needs have to be given charitably. This would be a direct conflict with what that individual wants for their life—living in the confines of what their religion is dictating. I heard in the Secret by Rhonda Byrne— "The Universe/God never tells you what you can or cannot have—the Universe only manifests in response to the request of the vibration stemming from your desires." So, if a person believes that they are created for poverty or mediocrity, then the Universe/God will only manifest what they believe and what they confess for their life. Consider this real situation of a married woman with two children and an abusive alcoholic husband. She is affiliated with a religious group whose name I will not disclose. Her dream is to put her two children through college, but she needs to finish school herself to better her financial position. Her husband has not held down a job in two years and is steadily putting her down for trying to do better. The woman wants to leave her husband, thinking she would accomplish more for herself and children if she was to leave him. But her church tells her that divorce is never an option and that if she proceeded with divorcing him—she would be in direct defiance against the church—and would consequently be excommunicated from the church. In a situation like this, how much liberty does this woman have in creating her own life when her emotional and spiritual support system fails her? So, what I am seeing in this real-life scenario is how religious practices can discourage a person from pursuing their God-given dreams. This is most definitely not the purpose of God indwelling us—so that we can be unproductive and unfulfilled?

Religion has become an addiction for many. Some people have become so caught up in doing good deeds for others that they often neglect the people that need them most—sometimes their own children, parents, or mates. After working in church ministries for more than thirty years, I have witnessed many pastor wives stray from their marriages, PKs (preachers' kids) getting into drugs and all kinds of forbidden activities, and becoming promiscuous—just to name a few. This by no means could be the work or the purpose of God—especially when family relationships are a high priority with God (at least according to the Bible).

The act of neglecting the need of family or even yourself for the sake of keeping religious practices is no different than that of a drug addict—who disregards the care of others so that he can get his "fix." All who are in close proximity to the drug addict will be affected negatively and will experience loss on some level. The same will be true for those who are religiously addicted—who disregard the cares of others to fulfill their religious dogma.

I am in no way bashing people who are religious, for I have my own personal rituals or religious acts that I do on a daily basis. But my objective is to bring awareness to people who are denouncing their own personal joy and happiness to fit into a ritualistic community. We should never make an effort to fit into any group at the cost of losing our individuality and happiness. We should seek associations with those who are in harmony with our personal beliefs—and not confine ourselves to systems that forces us to meet their expectations.

Many people today do not ascribe to being religious…, but spiritual. Spirituality involves the recognition of a feeling or sense or belief that there is something greater than one's self. It ascribes that there is something more to being human than sensory experience—and that the greater whole of which we are part is cosmic or divine in nature. To be spiritual simply means to believe in God or a higher Intelligence. To believe in a power or source that influences all of creation.

A spiritual person seeks the truth from a higher guidance from within his or her own *being* by sensing what's right and what's wrong. What is important is that humans gravitate to the understanding that all that is needed in inheriting the life meant for them resides in the intellect of the *inner self.* It is in the awareness of *self* that we rise to universal power—the power given to us by God. It is in our *inner self* that the mind of God is being understood on a day-by-day journey. When we open ourselves to the Universe—not bogged down with traditions and ancient religious mindsets—that the unfolding of truth becomes alive within us.

267

Let's not seek a set of rules and regulations given thousands of years ago to control the behavior of a predominantly superstitious group of people. However, let us seek the fresh words of wisdom that flow from a universal, loving, all-encompassing, non-judging energy. This energy is simply God, and it reflects the *essence* of who we are as human beings. We are God within ourselves, wrapped in human form, with multiple expressions, faces of every color, tongues of every language, personalities of all sorts, and gifts and callings of all kinds. We are called to the higher level of *self*—as collective individuals joined together to create one universal love.

Where religion dictates, wars will fester.

J. Meddling

Article 42

Heaven & Hell
(Literal or Mythical)

A question that I am frequently asked relating to religion is: "Is heaven & hell a literal place, or is it simply imaginary?" I am always cautious when answering questions that can only have an abstract answer. Abstract because no of us were there in the beginning when all things came into being. I am also cautious because the people who usually ask this question typically do not possess the fundamental knowledge of the Bible's developmental history for me to begin an intelligent dialogue.

One must understand the basics as to how the Bible came into existence and its many developmental processes before the authenticity of its words can be accepted as truth. Though I believe in the principles of the Bible, however, I also believe that much of the interpretation has been manipulated through time—by religious and political men to promote their own agendas. With that being said, we must also understand that the translation of what's perceived as "truth" has not been completely represented in the writing of the Bible. And once again, I do believe strongly in the basic principles of the Bible—principles that support love, peace, and goodwill toward all people.

I believe that the original manuscripts (not completely added to the King James Version Bibles) were written to give hope, direction and deliverance to a *perceived* fallen humanity. But once powerful and influential leaders saw how potent and powerful this written word was and how they could control people and manipulate historical facts—a lust for power and dominance entered the religious arena. As a result of powerful and influential people wanting to control societies—the Bible was rewritten many times as a tool or yoke of constraint. The Bible has been rewritten with major references left out. It was also used as a tool to manipulate the ignorant, the poor, the desperate, the disenfranchised, and the superstitious. These things may not have been the original intent—but in a nutshell, that is eventually what happened.

Anything that has the power to control, subdue or manipulate—will be used to do just that by opportunistic individuals. For example, many slaves who were brought from Africa were persuaded to become Christians. They were programmed to believe that in order to be a good Christian or follower of Christ—they had to be a faithful slave. The largest slave trade in the history of the world was created by Christian European nations. The **Atlantic slave trade** or **transatlantic slave trade** took place across the Atlantic Ocean from the 16th through the 19th century. The vast majority of slaves transported to the New World were Africans from the central and western parts of the continent, sold by Africans to European slave traders who then transported them to North and South America. The numbers were so great that Africans who came by way of the slave trade became the most numerous Old-World immigrants in both North and South America before the late eighteenth century. Consequently, many slaves lost their inherent identity to a European belief system—a gospel that was not at all "Good News" for the slaves. Many of the slaves converted to a religion that gave no reference to their native spirituality and showed no regard for their native history. They were then forced into the European customs, traditions, and belief systems even though the slave was considered no more than mere property. But forcing this new belief in hopes of slaves conforming to subordination made the slaves more manageable—because if you can change a person's belief about what's appropriate and inappropriate—you change their convictions which makes them compliant. Therefore, as a tool of manipulation to guilt slaves into servitude, often the term "hell" was used by religious/ Christian slave owners to motivate a slave's compliance. And if the fear of *hell* didn't convince them—the whip would. It was believed by the so-called "good" slave owners— to be more humane rather than beating a healthy and hard-working slave into submission. A healthy slave was more valuable to an owner than one that was beaten up and unable to work for several days. In the history of religion, brutish "slavers" and leaders' main objective was to isolate people from the knowledge of their heritage, to make them subjective and to exploit their skills. I am not a basher of religion and believe that there's nothing wrong with religion as long as it allows others to be free and to practice their worship freely. But when any religion is used to enslaves or imprisons either by way of physical captivity or emotional and psychological captivity—it is wrong. This is deemed no more than brutish manipulation.

What's crucial to understand is that high-ranking religious leaders like the Catholic Popes and the head of the universal college of bishops often have a political stake in society—and many unfortunately use their cloak of religion to control groups and cultures of people by fear and intimidation. This is not to suggest that Popes and bishops are innately evil—but understanding that institutions have their own agenda. And those who were/ are under such powers often feel that if they disregarded the laws or ordinances set by the established Powers—that they are in defiance to the laws of God. Without pointing the finger at any religious group, the early religious institutions and authorities, slaughtered many innocent people in the name of God—inferring that all who did not accept their belief as the authorized religion of God was an infidel and did not deserve to live. We see this same religious and political dominance in the Bible in Acts 9:1-30 with the Apostle Paul, who slew Christians in the name of Rome but later became converted to live for a God who represented love.

Now getting to the subject of "hell," I will make references to the Bible because most people in our western world are familiar with stories of hell from the Bible—even though other religions make references to hell. Most other religions speak of "hell" in some form or another, but they do not all believe "hell" to be a place of perpetual torment. Most religions do not use the word "hell" in reference to eternal retribution for wrongdoings. Mainly those who are of the Christian based faith believe in hell as a literal place where evildoers will burn forever for their non-repented sins, but this perspective is not shared with all of the major religions.

There are five "major" religions practiced in the world today, and they are Islam, Hinduism, Judaism, Buddhism, and Christianity. And only two religions from the five believe in a literal heaven and hell. These two religions that support the heaven & hell concept are Christianity and Islam. The word "hell" in the Bible is a mistranslation of the Hebrew word "Sheol," which means the "pit," better known as simply the "grave." Another mistranslation for the word hell found in the Bible is "Gehenna," known as the valley of the sons of Hinnom, where Israelites used to conduct abominable things like phallus worship (where they worshiped images of the male and female sexual organs) and committed human sacrifice, rituals where children ran through burning coals barefoot and etc. Later "Gehenna" became known as a literal dumping ground or junkyard. When Jesus used the term "hell," He was referring to Gehenna (a dumping ground or junkyard) symbolically as the place where things go to simply never exist again. My personal belief is that this is a metaphoric place signifying the abolishment of evil consciousness. Neither Jesus nor the Hebrew Bible, he interpreted, endorsed the view that departed souls go to paradise or everlasting pain. And unlike most Greeks, ancient Jews traditionally did not believe the soul could exist at all apart from the body. On the contrary, for them, the soul was no more than "breath." When Adam began as a lump of clay, then God "breathed" life into him, and he became a living being (Genesis 2:7). But when Adam stopped breathing or living, he was back to simply being a lump of clay— from ashes to ashes and dust to dust. And so, the Hebrew Bible itself assumes that the dead are simply dead and that the body simply lies in the grave and there's no consciousness ever again.

So, I believe that Jesus metaphorically referenced "hell" to the Israelites as a place where all the religious rhetoric, rituals, manipulations, and taking advantage of the poor would be laid to rest and forgotten—or, in other words, to be burned up and never seen again. This prediction, however, did come to pass around 67-70 AD when the Roman legions surrounded the city of Jerusalem and began to annihilate the Jewish stronghold. By the year 70 AD, the attackers had breached Jerusalem's outer walls and began a systematic neutralization of the city. The assault culminated in the burning and destruction of the Temple that served as the center of Judaism. I do not believe that Jesus was teaching a literal "hell" but was symbolically making reference to the demise of an abusive government that would be trampled beneath the earth—not to be remembered no more. I believe that "hell" is understood as the place for eternal suffering, it does not exist literally but exists metaphorically.

However, I do believe that hell's more literate meaning lies within the symbolism of a state of being—living in a state of perplexity, poverty, ignorance, sickness, or any other situation defining the discomforts of life. On a personal level, hell can be a mindset of destitution— "For as a man believes in his heart, so is he" (paraphrased). Proverbs 23:7—and Mathew 8:13 make a similar reference. However, religious leaders who intimidate others into converting to a particular faith do so by removing the symbolism of hell and making it into a literal hell—a place of perpetual punishment for those who violate the commandments or even the law of that day.

I believe that heaven—just like hell is also symbolic. When Jesus taught his disciples to pray in reference to heaven, it was with the anticipation that they would get the concept that heaven was within the human heart. Jesus taught his disciples to pray by saying, "...Thy kingdom come, thy will be done, on earth as it is in heaven" (Matthew 6:10 KJV). If the *perceived will of God* is done on earth, there would be no need to "go to heaven,"—for peace and harmony among mankind would be present, making this heaven on earth. I believe that Jesus, along with Buddha, Muhammad, and the many other ancient patriots for peace on earth, taught the same message that heaven is within the human heart and not somewhere distant out in space. It does not matter the terminology they used for heaven because their message was a message of human wholeness, which I interpret as heaven on earth.

We can and will experience heaven and hell here on earth, but it is totally our choice which reality we choose to live in. We create our beds of reality by our perception of what is.

All of the major religions mentioned, Hinduism, Buddhism, Judaism, Islam, and Christianity, all agree that there is a God or Higher Intelligence, but none of them totally agree on the other basics like:

1. The number of Deities (how many Gods there are)

2. God's gender

3. Reincarnation (life after death)

4. Nature of God (judgemental, benevolent, or neutral)

5. Path to salvation (good works, perfect karma, or Jesus)

6. Nature of the afterlife (heaven/hell, earth plane, or to exist as energy.)

When we heighten our consciousness and become aware that we are the expression of Higher Intelligence in human form, we will indelibly become the controller of our earthly experiences. We will make our experience on earth heavenly—and will bring unity to the world.

Article 43

Am I A Christian?

When I think of my friends and associates who profess Christianity, I am reminded of the diversities that lie within their individual beliefs. I once heard one of my Christian friends proclaiming to another mutual Christian friend—that they were not a "true" Christian. And their premise for making that statement was based on some of our friends' habits, characteristics, and form of worship. I was gravely shocked that a person would say such things about someone they had known for ten plus years. This was a Christian brother making this statement to another mutual brother—that we'd often sat and had dinner with in his home. I was hurt to know that he could so easily disqualify someone he'd known for so many years, from being a Christian—based on religious practices—he simply wasn't accustomed to.

As human beings, we grow up with different religious or ritualistic practices that we believe make us right with God. And sometimes people will unknowingly superimpose their ritualistic practices into our belief system and deem it as the authentic work and *will* of God. Every experience in our life makes an impression on our spirituality/ beliefs—whether we are conscious of it or not. There is no way for us to separate our life experiences from our spirituality—they are one. With that being said, I believe that all of life is spiritual—the good, the bad, and the ugly.

So, to answer the question—am I a Christian? Well, in most religious circles, I would be considered a Christian based on my behavior, religious practices and deeds. But I have come to a new reality of truth for myself that disconnects me from carrying any religious title. I consider myself one who live and walks in the awareness of God consciousness. If I allow myself to carry the title "Christian,"—then I subject myself to the proposed or expected behavior of others who are called by that title—even though being a Christian means being a follower of Christ. People will still subject you to their personal opinion of what "Christ-likeness" looks like. And, of course this is often their own perception and interpretation of Christ. So, if I call myself a Christian—I would be superimposed upon me to live the way others believe that I should live—and not be an expression of my own individuality. But isn't it written that the disciples where first called Christians in Antioch? See Acts 11:26 *and when he found him, he brought him to Antioch. So, for a whole year Barnabas and Saul met with the church and taught great numbers of people.* ***The disciples were called Christians first at Antioch*** (NIV). This scripture denotes that Paul and Barnabas who were expounding on the teaching of Jesus Christ—made such an impression upon the observers—that the observers are the ones who coined them with the title of Christians. My point is simply this; We do not need to wear or give ourselves a title to be known as *something*. All you have to do is simply live your life—and others can crown you with a title if that's important to you. Jeffrey Dahmer didn't give himself the title of being a serial killer and sex offender—his actions and the observers of his deeds gave him his title.

I have chosen not to be defined by other people's belief systems or religious practices—even though I have my own spiritual/ ritualistic practices. I have discovered that I am a potpourri of many organized religious belief systems—but with each of them, I disagree with one or more major aspects—which probably disqualify me as being "true" to any of them. I take from each belief system what I believe is right for me and leave the rest for someone else who might prefer it. I personally see religions like a huge buffet where you place on your tray the food that you like, and whatever you do not prefer is someone else's preference. However, I do not pick and choose what to believe based on its convenience for me. I simply choose what I believe based on what makes sense for practical and relevant living. **I see religion as an organized system that attempts to give meaning to our lives, where there is a supreme being that we call God., orchestrating everything**.

Some would say that God has only one salvation plan that's tied up into one religious' truth. I believe the Supreme Intelligence of the universe is too vast and too broad for one religion to embrace the wholeness of its deity. We cannot contain or understand all that consists of God according to the bible in Isaiah 55:8-9 *"For my thoughts are not your thoughts, nor are your ways my ways, says the Lord. For as the heavens are higher than the earth, so are my ways higher than your ways and thoughts than your thoughts."*

It is also my conviction that God, the Supreme Intelligence, abides proportionately in each and every person and is even disguised sometimes as the most heinous individual—at least heinous from the human perspective. We can only deem something "evil" if we are the creator of it. What I mean is that—to *proclaim* that a gun is evil—you would have to be the inventor of the gun with the understanding of the gun's intentions. We do not know the Creator's intention for any one in particular. Therefore, we cannot rightly call anyone "evil." Only the Creator can—who knows the intention behind the creation. To further my point—I am inclined to believe that we are all mere actors on this stage called life—and that our roles are *somewhat* pre-determined—or more accurately **pre-known**. Such is the case of Judas who betrayed Jesus. Theologians have agreed that Judas Iscariot was predestined (pre-chosen) to be Jesus' betrayer—and I am of the same inclination, having researched and studied the scriptures. In the bible, it reads concerning Judas:

In the evening He came with the twelve. Now as they sat and ate, Jesus said, "Assuredly, I say to you, one of you who eats with Me will betray Me." And they began to be sorrowful, and to say to Him one by one, "Is it I?" And another said, "Is it I?" He answered and said to them, "It is one of the twelve, who dips with Me in the dish. **The Son of Man indeed goes just as it is written of Him, but woe to that man by whom the Son of Man is betrayed!** *It would have been good for that man if he had never been born."* Mark 14:17-21 NKJV

Now getting back to the topic about my identification with Christianity. For the largest portion of my life, I have identified with being a Christian—but I no longer aim to fulfill a title or to be pigeon-holed into religious expectations. I currently live intentional and is keenly devoted to my purpose. I am more profoundly governed by my awareness of living in observance of my own convictions. I live reverently to the God who lives and speaks within the confines of my subconscious. My lifestyle is one that most people would consider respectful and honorable. I am proud of who I am—and striving to grow to my highest level of awareness. I Am Indeed Free!

Article 44

What Is Prayer

As children, many of us were given words to recite as a prayer—for instance: "*Now I lay me down to sleep...*" or "*God is love, God is good, let us thank Him for our food.*" These are what I consider as stencils for prayer. Most of us are taught to pray to a God who is perceived to be out in space or far away in heaven. I believe that the God of the universe is presently abiding within our human vessels—our bodies. When we understand that God is never away from us—we will find ourselves empowered with the confidence that our prayers are always heard and answered.

Prayer has been given such complexity that many feel that praying is futile and that only "holy people" are heard. Many believe that there is a certain way to pray or that they have to be bowed down on their knees in order for the prayer to be genuine. None of this, of course, is true. Much of this erroneous thinking has derived from the religious pictures of people kneeling with folded hands—that we've seen from childhood. We have been inundated with the idea that we must carry out certain rituals in order to be heard by God. Even pictures of a muscular God reaching down from heaven and touching the fingertip of a mere mortal man are all depictions of humans existing in a spiritually fallen state—in need of redemption. We have also seen the "Footstep in the Sand" pictures giving us the perception that God is some obscured entity invisibly lingering around, waiting to carry us when we get weak. It is a reassuring thought that there is someone who will help us when we are too weak to carry our burden. But the perception lends to this fallacy that God is outside of us.

We must become aware that there is no one in particular—to bow down to, though many believe that this humble position shows reverence to Higher Intelligence. But I believe that true reverence is walking in the awareness or consciousness that God is in you and that you are in God—and the two of you are one. There is no separation of human beings and the Creator God. Human beings, alone with all of creation—are expressions of God in material form. This is why Jesus repeated in St. John 14:19, saying (paraphrased) that "*I am in the Father (God) and the Father is in me, and we are one.*" Jesus also proclaims in prayer that his disciples become one with the Father (God) even as He (Jesus) is one with God. Being one with God is simply a matter of understanding that God resides within our human frames. The Creator speaks to us directly through and *from* our subconscious mind, which many identify as our spirit. It is to the subconscious mind, spirit or the *inner self* that we pray—and not outside of ourselves. This is because God exists within us to communicate with us. So, when we beseech God (by way of prayer), we are simply

284

tuning-in to the voice of our subconscious mind or *inner spirit*. This is why the Bible says that "... *it is God who is at work within you, both to will (desire) and to do His good pleasure*" (Philippians 2:13.) So, your *inner self* (the place where God abides in you) already knows better than your conscious mind the things you need and desire most. Therefore, it is unnecessary to continuously ask for the same thing over again—unless your repetition helps you achieve the level of belief where positive emotions flow. And I clearly understand that sometimes it takes repetition to help us connect our faith—but once faith has been established—the only thing needed for manifestation is expectancy. When faith is actuated—the conscious mind can relax in knowing that the request is on the way. It is a fact that sometimes we lose hope or faith in the things we're believing for—if it takes too long to manifest. It then becomes necessary to *request again* as a means of reestablishing our intentions, focus, and energy on the things desired.

So, prayer should not be a ritual we do in order to get into God's good graces, but it is an encounter with our own *God-like* potential. Prayer can also be understood as the expansion of our human creativity or the reestablishing of *self* to the infinite power found within our own being.

The final misrepresentation about prayer is that prayer is a way of softening the heart of God and bringing ourselves to a level of worthiness. Nothing is further from the truth, in my opinion. We are not here on earth to try and become worthy for heaven but to simply live out our creative abilities like the Higher Intelligence residing within us. Humans are the expressions of God—who are having an earthly experience where we are attempting to manifest our God-potential through our everyday lives. We are collectively the expressions of the Universal Intelligence. There is no higher plain than that of awareness of our own divinity. So let us live our lives like the kings and queens we were created to be— walking with our heads high, knowing that our very existence is confirmation of the elect calling into worthiness and wonder.

God is as connected to you - as salt is to the sea.

J. Meddling

Article 45

Where Does Personal Convictions Come From?

Why do we have convictions or consciousness of right and wrong? Where does this awareness come from? How does it relate or connect to our *sense of self*?

Almost every individual has an awareness of what's appropriate and inappropriate. Our concept of right and wrong stems from our childhood development. It later becomes our inner convictions after years of programming. Sometimes these inherent belief systems become challenged with new information as we evolve as spiritual beings. When we evolve to the level of consciousness that reminds us that we, in essence, are divine beings—it is then that we encounter conflict about what we've been taught as appropriateness. What I'm attempting to convey is that when we were children, our parents taught us what was right and wrong. They taught us what appropriate and inappropriate behavior was. This teaching or gathering of information throughout our life formed our convictions as adults about what was right and wrong. But as adults, our spiritual senses developed, and we began to apply critical thinking skills. We began to challenge the rationale behind our *inherited* convictions. We begin to ask ourselves; *why do I believe what I believe?* This crossroad is where the conflict about what we had accepted as being true or factual is now being put through the critical thinking process. As a result, we began to readjust our belief system, which inadvertently changed our personal convictions. Because of this conversion in *thinking*, what we once thought was wrong or *sinful* is no longer something we have negative emotions or convictions about. This is the actuation of our divinity at work. And I know that there may be readers thinking that human beings don't possess Divinity…only God is Divine. But I challenge you with the fact that God is as much you—as the impressions you have about yourself. What I mean is—our life as humans have been dulled and desensitize by programming that did not come from our Creator. The God of the universe lives and abides in each one of us. That makes us divine!

There is never a separation of God from us, no matter our behavior—because we always feel convictions which is indication that God is present. The Bible says, *"For in him (God) we live, and move, and have our being; as certain of your own poets have perfectly stated, for we are God's offspring"* (Acts 17:28). And if are indeed the offspring of God—then why would our Creator be interested in playing hide-and-seek with us by being allusive and unobtainable? God perfectly places *"Itself"* into our human frames so that we are always connected to divinity. So, the attributes of God are always abiding within us—even if we choose to behave otherwise. But if we are to live in prosperity and productively—tapping into those creative attributes is simply a matter of tuning in to the spirit of God. **And because this has to become a VERY intentional act—many will not grasp it.**

Our personal convictions serve as a guiding force, protecting the moral essence of who we are. For example, Judy believes that cheating on taxes is wrong, but her friend Sherry says to her that "*the government is always taking advantage of honest taxpayers, so you shouldn't feel bad claiming loss from your business that you really didn't incur—people do it all the time.*" But Judy declines the advice of her friend because Judy does not want to deal with feeling guilty about harboring a lie on her taxes. And she's afraid that if she gets audited—she won't be able to prove her losses.

This is an example of a personal conviction protecting the moral essence of an individual. Refusing to do what one believes to be wrong to maintain a level of inner peace is the reality of living in the awareness of Godliness—or simply living with a clear conscious. If Judy had taken the advice of her friend Sherry, Judy would have violated her own personal convictions, leaving her to feel wounded in her perception of *self*. This is why many people seek the advice of others concerning their own personal matters. They have violated their own conscious so many times that they become marred with guilt—which translates to confusion. Confusion become emotional clutter—and now this individual no longer trust their own decision making because they are not clear-headed. This kind of *guilty clutter* distances them from the inherited wisdom of God. In the story of the Garden of Eden, it was guilt that caused Adam to distance himself from God. Even if you do not believe the Garden of Eden story—consider the child who took a cookie from the cookie jar after the parent told them not to. The disobedient child, as a result of feeling guilty for their disobedience, shelters in their room to prevent facing the parent. The story of Adam hiding from God after eating from the forbidden tree—reflects the behaviors of human beings when they feel shame for doing something wrong. And when we isolate ourselves from our own source—then where can we go to be restored? Just like the child who hides from the parent because of disobedience—will at some point return to their source (the parent) for provision. But there will be a lack of confidence when that child request something again of the parent—because of the guilt factor. This is what I'm referring to as *guilty clutter*!

Another example of this is when you loan someone some money, and they do not pay you back within the time agreed upon. Often the borrower has the tendency to avoid you—right? The shame or guilt of not having what is owed causes them to shun you. People who continuously violate their own convictions—often become dulled and out-of-tune with the voice of their inner conscious—thereby silencing the instructing voice of God. So, when they pray to God, they cannot recognize the *voice* of God because of the chatter of guilt. Instead of hearing the *voice* or instructions of God—all they hear is the condemning voice within themselves, saying *they do not deserve to receive anything*. The *voice* or instructions of God is heard and understood through our inner consciousness. When we disarm the voice of our inner conscious because of our *perceived* unworthiness—we falter in getting the instructions we need for our lives. To put it another way—not following your inner convictions is denouncing the God force abiding within you.

We should never behave outside of our moral belief system. Since there is such a diversity of beliefs and standards among human beings, one should live by their own convictions and not the conviction of another. Neither should we judge the conviction and belief systems of others, for there is multiformity in life experiences, which mode every person's belief. And as I stated earlier—how and what we believe is based upon everything we've been taught and what we have experienced. Therefore, we cannot rightly judge a person's experiences—and just as we reserve judgment of another person's experiences—neither should we judge their beliefs.

Article 46

I Want To Be Free
(Don't Confine Me by Defining Me)

Many people adopt religious titles to define who they are and what they believe. They wear these titles as badges of honor—while others become caught up in the status of being a part of a certain religion to give themselves a sense of identity. For example, they may take on the titles or stance of being a Christian, Muslim, Buddhist, Hindu, or Jew (in relation to Judaism.) And there is absolutely nothing wrong with having religious beliefs—in fact, we all believe in something that we deem sacred to us. We may not necessarily wrap it in the cloak of religion, but we all have a code of conduct that we live by—whether it's bad or good. But if the objective of having a religion is solely based upon having an identity for the sake of being accepted—or to fit into a clan or group—then there needs to be a serious evaluation of that motive. I personally believe that if we are going to follow any set of rules or regulations in a religion—it should first make sense to us. Secondly, we should wholeheartedly believe in it. Thirdly, it should be inclusive or available to all people, or else it will be no different than being in a fraternity, sorority, or club. Fourthly, and this is only my personal appeal—but it should be a belief system that elevates the human race and not just a selected few. I have long believed since I was a young adult that every human on earth has a part to play in the stage of life to make the world around us a better place to live in. As far as we *really* know—we only get one shot at this reality that we now exist in. Oh…there may be other realities that far extend this *one* existence—but for sure, we have this reality at hand. And it is my contingency that we make the most meaningful impression upon the lives that we are able to touch—including our own.

Religious Creeds

I believe that if we live by religious creeds to simply obtain what we *perceive* as an escape from an eternal doom or to be a part of an impressive sector—then our belief might be in vain. If our religion is not inclusive to all or requires us to shun those who might be considered undesirables—might our religion be confining and defining a behavior that does not exemplify unity? And what I mean by becoming confined and defined by religion is that we become pigeonholed into a certain expectation of conduct that we might have trepidation in believing. But because we have placed ourselves under a particular religious title—there's no wiggle room for allowances. Our religion may deed or demand certain conduct, deed, or response to any given situation that we may not be in total agreement with. In other words, we are not given the room to deviate from the religious protocol—except we risk straying away from what we say we believe. An example of this is found in the bible when

Jesus encounters the woman who was caught in adultery. In St. John 8: 1-11, a woman was caught committing adultery by the Pharisees who were the religious leaders and the scribes who were lawyers. These preachers and lawyers' came to Jesus while he was teaching at the temple—and their motive was to trap Jesus by getting him to denounce Moses Law relating to a person being caught in adultery. They wanted Jesus to condemn this woman and have her to be stoned to death, which was the punishment by law if such a person was caught in the act. There are many interesting facts—the first being how merciless the religious leaders were toward this woman. The second aspect is: why wasn't the man who was caught committing the act of adultery with the woman not brought out to be stoned as well? The law in the Old Testament or Torah of Leviticus 20:10 states that both parties should be put to death in such an act. But Jesus steps outside of the religious law and simply states in St. John 8: 7 *He who is without sin among you; let him cast the first stone.* And by answering in this manner— no one could claim that Jesus went against the Mosaic Law—which was the intent of the Pharisees and scribes. And though Jesus did not refute the Mosaic Law, his act of mercy towards the woman was not what the religious law deemed. Jesus did not give in to his "haters"—being the Pharisees and scribes—the preachers and the lawyers.

My point is this—following religious protocols like the Pharisees & scribes—might lure you from showing mercy—when mercy is needed. But focusing on what is right and best for your fellowman should become our focus when following religious creeds—just as Jesus exemplified with the woman caught in adultery. It is because of this kind of contention that comes from organized religion—that I choose to be free from religious titles, expectations, and confinements. I choose not to be defined as a righteous human being based on religious characterization. I choose to be free-spirited, free-thinking, and free from being categorized. However, I do not believe that this gives me a license to do whatever I want. I am, yet, strongly carried by my convictions to present myself in a respectful and loving manner to everyone I encounter. I believe and live by the Golden Rule of *doing unto others as you would have them do unto you.* I also believe in extending mercy to others—as I would want mercy extended to me.

Be What You Preach

If our identity is encapsulated in the religious titles we wear—then there must also be a lifestyle that stands in congruency with our beliefs. As Texans say *...all hat and no cattle* is the same reference to what the bible says *... faith without works is dead.* We shouldn't just talk the talk...but also ...walk the walk. I have seen where religious people will bend, alter and even denounce aspects of what they proclaim to believe just to fit into their agenda, lifestyle, or in any manner that will best serve them. I believe this to be the reason for so many non-religious individuals becoming disenchanted with organized religion...because of this hypocrisy.

Those who confess and identify themselves with the association of any religion are thereby subjected to the expectations and disciplines of that belief system. And there is absolutely nothing wrong with having an ideology that serves as your moral compass. In fact, I have my own moral compass that's not necessarily tied to any religion—but govern by an intuitive nature of what's right or wrong.

Human Nature Hates Confinement

I personally believe that the intuitive nature or God aspect...in all human beings seeks to be free from the confinement of ideologies that do not *naturally* guide us. I also believe this to be the reason for the inability to *consistently* keep commandments, follow the rules, adhere to, abide by, or remain constant to creeds. Human nature does not particularly like restraints. And yes, I understand that there must be rules and laws in place in order to have a civil society—but many human struggles in keeping religious creeds are internal issues of self-control. We often try and control things internally that are not meant to be controlled. One simple example of this is those who take a vow of celibacy to serve God. This sacrificing of a natural human desire in order to be more connected to God, in my humble opinion, is a shipwreck waiting to happen—especially if a person does not possess the *natural* inclination to live this kind of life. And as I have stated throughout this book—there is no way we can become separated from the Highest Intelligence. Being closely connected to the Highest Intelligence is a matter of tuning in with all of your heart, mind, and strength. And one does not have to live a life of celibacy in order to do this.

I mentioned a moment ago in the above paragraph that our intuition *naturally* guides us. There is a *natural law* that dictates human behavior without anyone telling you that something is right or wrong. For example, a child does not need instructions on how to lie because it is innate in all human beings. Better yet, that same child does not have to be taught how to feel ashamed after being caught in that lie. Shame and guilt are also innate. Just as we have the "Law of the Land" to keep us sensitive to the rights of our fellow man—we innately have a *natural law* that guides our conscious toward the sensitivity for our fellow man. In basic terms, we do not have to be taught to be good or to do right by others. Of course, we understand that in our society, we have people with psychological and emotional imbalances who require correction—whereby we need the Law of the Land to intervene by way of enforcement. But the majority of us are innately aware of how to be good to one another. And whether we are conscious of this fact or not—human beings would rather live from this *natural* place of conviction. We do not require religion to tell us how to be kind to one another. I am also of the opinion that living a life of goodwill towards all people should not be a task for those who live authentically. When we live authentically, we do not put on an act for others to be impressed by. We allow ourselves to be *comfortable in our own skin,* and we interact in truth. When we live authentically, we focus on connections with others and not possessions. We should live humbly and embrace the imperfections. This way of thinking and living prevents us from being reactive to things we disagree with. It teaches us how to be responsive—rather than reactive.

Confusion in Organized Religion

The confusion that often comes with people of the same religion having various interpretations is another reason why many have become disenchanted with organized religion. The chaos, confusion, and debates about translations among people of the same faith become unattractive to any potential convert. Not having clear lines of references on a belief becomes problematic when trying to convince someone about the religion you associate yourself with. And the scattered interpretations between people of the same religious organization are what I believe to be the result of various people relating God from their own personal experiences. But the fullness of *whom or what* God is cannot be explained or isolated to our human experience alone. People create an image of their *perceived* interactions with God and deem it as truth. And this is how organized religion ends up with confusion in its belief system. I talked about this very point in article 43 **Am I A Christian?**

Over the years, I have observed religious people feuding over trivial things relating to ceremonial practice and ordinances. There are...and have always been religious wars over territory—where religious groups who all claim to love God are fighting for the "so-called" cause of God. There are disagreements among religious folks about what foods are Kosher and what are not. And there are so many other meaningless disharmonies over things that have nothing to do with elevating the human race. After all, shouldn't religion be more about building bridges with humanity rather than burning them down? Shouldn't there be more of a focus on our commonalities as human beings rather than focusing on the differences between us?

We witness a lot of religious chaos because people hold their own morals, values, and belief system above others. But none of *them or us* has a monopoly on what is *absolutely* right or wrong concerning another's beliefs and values. In order to understand the *absolute* truth about any given thing—one would have to know what was—or is, in the mind of our Creator. And since none of us was there at the beginning of creation—we cannot know what the absolute intention of our Creator is. At best, we can live out of a place of harmony with ourselves and with all people—and maybe in doing so, we will manifest the intentions of our Creator through our love for one another. We might find ourselves becoming more accepting of others' religious expressions if we change our focus.

My opinion is that it takes all of humanity working in one consciousness to possibly embody the *mind* of God. When we work as one people with a united mind—we'll begin to see and understand the truth, purpose, and fullness of all things. Perhaps, we can collectively unfold the relevancy and *personhood* of God in our lives and in this world when we become united as the human race.

Once You Define Me

Once you define me—you confine me. We cannot thrive as co-creators with God when we are confined to human expectations. Once we are given a title or label, we become restricted to a perceived behavior that consequently revokes our ability to be free-spirited. Jesus himself had to refuse the expectations of those who thought that He should become their king after feeding five thousand people with five loaves of bread and two small fish. They wanted to confine Jesus to a title because of the great miracle he'd performed by feeding the multitude. But Jesus understood that a title was not what he needed in order to do the work of serving his fellow man. If He had succumbed to their expectations of becoming king—the people would have always seen him as their source. But Jesus wanted the people to know that they had to become their own source. That's precisely why Jesus asked his disciple Philip *"Where shall we buy bread to feed all these people?"* (St. John 6:5). Jesus put the responsibility of feeding the people into the hands of everyday people like Philip. Jesus was conveying that you are kings and queens among yourselves. You can be your own providers if you would just look around and use what is at hand…like the five loaves of bread and two fish. The miracle they were looking for was already at their disposal. Jesus did not want to be the "only" orchestrator of miracles—but wanted the people and his disciples to orchestrate their own miracles. The same potential Jesus had to multiply food was the same potential that lay dormant in his disciples—and in you. So, Jesus did not want to be recognized as a king, because being their king meat being a kind of provider. They would have always been dependent upon him to make their life comfortable—just like many people today depend on a well-fare system. (See St. John 6:1-15). Being a king would have confined Jesus to the people's expectations—and they would have never ventured to become self-reliant. So true is the saying: *"If you give a man a fish, you will feed him for the day. If you teach a man to fish, you feed him for a lifetime."*

There is absolutely nothing wrong with being *defined* and *confined* as long as we understand the responsibility that comes with that label. We must also be willing to be under the scrutiny of those who hold us accountable. We should, however, know whether or not this is our season to handle the potential aggressions of people with contrasting opinions or views—just as Jesus knew His season to be acknowledged as king. Every leader should be mindful of the influence they have on others. And even though every mature and independent thinker should take responsibility for themselves—many, however, do not.

Influence & Example

We who are strong must indeed help bear the infirmity of the weak. This statement relates not only to the religious folks—but to our community as a whole on a state and national level as well. And it is unfortunate that many of our state and national leaders forget this basic premise of leadership. Just maybe, this basic premise is forgotten because there is such a lack of accountability to the very citizens who appointed or voted these leaders into these positions. Those who are considered "strong" and the pillars of our communities—are doing a great disservice to communities when they fail to exhibit morality in their leadership. After all, isn't this what we expect of those that we put in charge of our communities, states, and nation? We hold our leaders to a higher standard than we sometimes hold ourselves to. But we understand as a society that this responsibility of good moral representation comes with the territory of the job or position. And this is exactly why when a leader or any influential individual is caught doing something that is morally questionable—we show little mercy in ridiculing and criticizing them. The label that one wears carries a lot of responsibilities and expectations.

Seeing that no person is faultless—having labels and titles will not eradicate our imperfections. And though most reasonable people understand this—we still judge harshly those in leadership who betray our trust. But this is because we propose our morality and expectations of others. The title or label carries the weight of responsibility—and that responsibility demands perfection…at least from our human expectations. I believe that many of these expectations are unrealistic for anyone to perfectly achieve. However, I am not advocating living without moral restraints because I strongly believe that leaders and people in "power" should be held to a higher standard because they have chosen to be in the spotlight of ridicule and scrutiny. However, I do believe that we should always stay focused on being true to our own convictions—and not allowing ourselves to be devastated by the actions of others. We should always be true to ourselves and be responsible for our own lives. I have heard many great athletes state that they are not trying to be anyone's "role model." Their consensus is the idea of not trying to live up to others' expectations. The thought of trying not to fail anyone's expectations is more responsibility than anyone should have to bear. It is not likely that any of us can suit the need and expectations of others and maintain our own sense of freedom.

Confined and Defined in Relationships

As this subject relates to relationships—there are huge dynamics in how people are labeling (or not labeling) their relationships. I am hearing more people in relationships say that they want to be free from the traditional expectations and titles that typically define relationships. They are not seeking to be free from the relationship—but not wanting to have a title such as a husband or a wife, boyfriend or girlfriend connected to them. Around the world, people are redefining relationship dynamics that do not require a title. People often use the phrase *It's Complicated* in relation to a relationship that doesn't have a clear title.

I also personally know of married couples who live in separate houses and who are very content with this arrangement (usually couples in their 40s and up). And what about "open marriages," where a couple agrees to have other sexual partners with one another's consent? We can see how the dynamics of traditional titles and expectations in relationships have also changed.

Though I am not endorsing or advocating any of these arrangements, I cannot help but realize that people are attempting to maintain their personal identity by not allowing themselves to be confined to cultural norms or by the expectations of others. And if we choose not to be confined to others' expectations, then let's not harness ourselves to titles and labels. We should live our lives to our own expectations and enjoy being the free spirit we innately are.

Article 47

Understanding *Self* in the Family Unit
(Tribute to my family)

I am warmly reminded of my childhood days as a seven-year-old boy who was awakened on school mornings—by the aroma of bacon and eggs, pancakes and oatmeal being prepared. It was always the smell of breakfast cooking that would wake me and my six siblings—signifying that it was time to get up and prepare for school. My mother would awaken before sunrise to prepare a breakfast fit for a king's table—and the royalties being my father and six siblings. Not only did she arise early to prepare breakfast, but made sure that we got our dose of cod liver oil—which was chased with a glass of orange juice. My mother would line us up like little soldiers to give us our daily dose of the cheapest cold and flu prevention known during the sixties. She would see us off to school one by one with a kiss on each of our cheeks. Not only would she see us off, but she would be waiting on the porch or at the front door when we came home from school. I did not think about it as a child, but thinking back on those moments as an adult, it was always an assuring feeling to come home and seeing mother smiling on the porch. It was as if she had been waiting all day for our return from school. There was always a treat to come home to. Again, the meal would already be on the kitchen table—steaming hot. Mother always validated my siblings and me with the love that she showed in her everyday routine of caring for us.

As a young boy growing up with a severe speech impediment and learning disorder, my mother would encourage me by saying, *"one day, you will rule the world."* What she really meant was that one day I would not be dictated by my inadequacies and that I would rise above the disappointments of being a slow learner. As a child, those words continuously rang in my soul. Today, I am no longer haunted by the fears of inadequateness of speech or stuttering—for the reality of my *higher self* or the God in me came alive through my mother's encouragement. As an adult, I still hear the voice of God through my mother's words. My sense of *self* and awareness of God is a direct manifestation of my mother's encouragement. Little did I know then that in this small house full of so much love and encouragement would come the introduction to me learning *wholeness*.

The small three bedroom and one-bath house that gave shelter to seven children and two parents always embodied the fresh scent of pine-sol and lemon-scented furniture polish. Though we were poor by society's standards, we felt like the richest kids on earth. As a matter of fact, we as children didn't even know that we were classified as poor—because we had both mother and father in the home that showed their affection to us as well as to one another. I fondly remember my mother and father playfully wrestling with each other on the living room floor and my siblings and I watching and laughing hysterically. We were wondering who would win the wrestling match between mom and dad because mom was a farm girl raised with three brothers and knew how to rough-house with the best of them. My father, on the other hand, was a small man—much smaller than my mother. Often mother won the wrestling match... But I assumed daddy let her win. I also remember the family outings at the lake where mother had already prepared lunches for all the children, and daddy had the duty of getting the fishing poles ready to catch the fish that we would later have for dinner. We would spend the whole day outside, entertained by the simple unity of our family. In those days, it did not take much for children to have fun.

I remember how my father would take the family out for entertainment which was no more than a car ride around the town usually. I was about five or six, and daddy would take the family riding because we didn't have the money to go to an amusement park— so our recreation was just riding around in the car. I would stand on the back seat and make animated sounds when he turned the car sharply around corners. Scurrrrr...was the sound I made around every sharp turn. This was before children had to be buckled with seatbelts. I never told my daddy, but that was one of my favorite recreations.

And how about the time—when I was around seven, and he took the family fishing, and I was afraid to bate my hook? I did not know that he was aware of my fear of bating the worm onto the hook, but he gently took my fishing pole and, with a confident smile, hooked the worm so that I could fish with the older siblings. I did not tell my father, but that day he was my hero.

And I remember a few years later when daddy told me to stop throwing rocks at the birds early one Sunday morning. I was only eight, standing beside the family car, waiting for the rest of the family to come out and load up for church. But when my father went into the house to gather the rest of the family for church, I threw that last rock anyway and wounded a baby bird. I had hoped that daddy wouldn't see or hear the little bird in the bushes flopping and screeching in agony. But he did and asked me, "Why did you hit that innocent baby bird?" All I could answer was, "I don't know." Instead of whipping me like I thought he would, daddy made me watch that baby bird suffers as my punishment. The poor wounded baby bird, unable to fly or stand, screeched hysterically until it came to a diminishing weak chirp and finally died. I never told my dad, but that was the worst punishment that I could have ever gotten. And I never told him how that on that day—it made me appreciative of all life—even little birdies.

At the age of twelve, when I joined my first church, and as I nervously walked down the church aisle—I remember the proud look that my dad gave me. I did not tell him, but the look on his face gave me validation as a young man. On that day, I felt confident in making my own decisions.

Around age fourteen, I came to my father confused about the interpretation of a Bible verse. Though dad was busy doing upholstery, which he was always preoccupied with to make extra money to support our family—but being the great father he was—daddy put his hammer down, sat on a stool facing me, and took the time to explain in detail the meaning of that scripture. My father has always been an excellent teacher. I did not tell him, but I knew in that moment that one day, I too would be a great teacher of the Bible just like him.

Daddy was a fix-it-man too. I remember when the water heater went out, and he decided to replace it himself—knowing that it was a potentially dangerous job for a first-timer. But he took the challenge and replaced it himself. We all left the house except for mother when he turned on the power to the unit. We trusted that he knew what he was doing—but just in case...

And how about the time the roof was leaking—and to save money that we did not have to spend, daddy took on a roof repair single-handedly. Yeah, he fell through the roof with his legs dangling through the kitchen ceiling, hanging over mother's pot of soup that was cooking on the stove. But daddy fixed that roof by himself! I never told him, but seeing how he would take on projects and complete them—he assured me that I would one day be a "fix-it man" too.

When I was only sixteen, I remember coming to my father feeling ashamed and disappointed with myself as I announced to him that I had gotten a young woman pregnant and that I would soon be a father. I saw the disappointment on his face but heard the firm encouragement in daddy's voice when he said to me, *"Men in this family take care of their responsibilities."* Though I was young, I perfectly understood that I had placed myself in a man's position and that I could no longer live the life of a boy. The real-life experience of raising a child was now my new reality. I did not tell him, but I knew that day, because of his encouraging words, that I would be the best father I could be.

It has been through the support of my family unit, the portrayed strength of my father, and the nurturing love of my mother, who has now transitioned from this life—that has made me the man I am today. I learned to show compassion to all people through the compassion I saw my parents show to others. I have seen my parents bring in strangers from off the street and sit them down at our dinner table. I fondly remember how my mother not only made special treats for my siblings and me but for the neighborhood kids as well. She was affectionately called "The Pie Lady" by the children in our community. I learned to have an appreciation for all God's people and even God's creatures through the lesson my father taught me when I killed the baby bird with the rock. When I reflect back on that experience of killing that bird—it shows me how so many people suffer affliction as a result of another's pleasure, sport, or vindictiveness. I learned to value all life and to bear others' opinions and lifestyles—no matter how different it is from my own. I learned from my mother how to nurture the human soul and how all life blossoms when watered with love. I learned from her that no person is a waste of time. With my learning disability and speech impediment as a child, my mother validated me and assured me with her smile and touch that I could accomplish anything. She always looked at me so proudly—and through her eyes, I found confidence.

The simplistic love of the family unit has become a waned reality—with our busy lives and high-tech toys—that absorbs all of our attention from family. Maintaining the family as a unit is an "art" because it takes the creativity of loving parents to nurture the intricate balance of wholeness in a child. Our inner constitution or the convictions that we own—is first established by the influences of our parents in our early childhood years. I now understand that the subconscious influences (the influences of our childhood that we may not remember) are manifest in the behavior that we display as adults. Our understanding of our *inner self*—the place where God dwells, is primarily formed by the perception of those who influenced us as children. Simply speaking—we see or understand God through the eyes of our parents, teachers, and mentors. I believe people become who they are by the words spoken to them from their *influencers*. I now clearly understand that our self-awareness is delicately balanced on the impression that we project to others as well as their impression projected onto us. That is to say, the confidence we carry is because of how we see ourselves through the eyes of others. We are creatures who thrive on feeling accepted by those we admire, respect, and simply love. This is why the family unit is so crucial to an individual finding human wholeness. Because parents who nurture their children—as a result are teaching their children to be nurturers to the world.

There is no greater influence in our lives than the influence of the family unit—no matter the dynamics of the family. This is the foundation of all future potential. The influence of the family is where birth is given to our belief systems. Our belief system is what anchors us to our inner convictions. Therefore, let us appreciate the expressed love of God manifested in the family unit.

A nation is as strong as the families it embodies.

J. Meddling

Article 48

Who or What is God
(My Personal Belief)

This article will be my most challenging one to write because of the potential controversy around the "God Questions" in general. But like almost everyone else who has an opinion or belief of/ or in God—we hold very strong convictions to that belief. And right off the bat, let me state "as a matter of fact," nothing that I say in this article is absolute or law. But neither do I believe that out of the five major religions in the world, Islam, Judaism, Christianity, Buddhism, and Hinduism—hold the unadulterated truth or knowledge of who or what God is.

I do, however, believe in a God that is the Creator of all, an intelligent mind, the Source, and a "Predestinator" of every living thing. I believe that every living creature, whether micro or macro, small or large, visible or invisible, was created or birth from an intelligent source with a purpose and a plan. And even if that plan or purpose is not completely understood by finite minds or mere human intellect—this thing or entity that we call God is the mastermind behind it all. I believe it is quite evident, even in nature, that the intelligent source that I call God is the author of all the beauty that we behold when we see the trees and the stars and the innumerous creatures that walk and walk upon this earth. Even when we behold the bumblebee that modern-day science says shouldn't be able to fly because of its body dynamics—but yet the bumblebee keeps right on flying despite its odd body shape and small wings. And what about when we look at the variety of animals and plants in all of their beauty and splendor, with their unique instinct for survival. Could one not believe that an intelligent mind or source is behind all of this? Well, many reading this article might be saying to themselves; plants, animals, and even human beings are no more than present-day manifestations of evolution. This is to say that every living thing has simply evolved into what we now see—and that we do not need the concept of God to factor in the process of evolution. If human beings are simply the result of evolution—then our brains are no more than a random collection of chemicals such as serotonin, dopamine, glutamate, norepinephrine, and Gamma-aminobutyric acid. How can we then trust anything that we think or understand as human beings if we are simply the result of evolution?

Some might even believe that evolution, in fact, is this *thing* we call God. But I politely disagree with that opinion too, because in order for there to be an evolution, there has to be *something*, to begin with. There at least has to be a seed or an egg in order to construct any form of life—at least from a scientific perspective. And if you have a seed or an egg, then what gives that matter (seed & egg) the life or energy to become a living matter or organism? I humbly believe this is where the intelligent mind or God factors into the equation. I believe there has to be a supremely intelligent mind behind creation—and that life is not left to "chance" through evolution.

God as Energy, Spirit, and Life

Though I do not believe in *every* aspect of any holy book, I do value and appreciate the references that are made about God in these holy books as a means to having some form of foundation about where creation came from and how it began. So, I reference the bible in making this point since most people are familiar with the "story of creation." So, from Genesis 1:1-31, *In the beginning, God created...* The intelligent mind or God needed physical matter—a seed or egg in order to *infuse* life into it because matter by itself is non-living. The seed or egg could not on its own make itself alive or living in order to evolve. Life, Spirit, or energy (whichever you prefer to call it) is the only thing, in my opinion, that has the ability to evolve. A seed or an egg in a jar will never amount to anything other than what it is—even if left in that container for a million years. It is the energy, Spirit, or life that gives meaning and purpose to matter. And I believe that this thing we call God is the source that gives all living things the ability to live, breathe, think, and evolve. Without the intelligent mind of God infusing "itself" into matter—no life would exist that does exist.

317

How Physics Explains God

The existence of an intelligent source, an infinite mind, or God can be explained in physics. Though physics was a subject I struggled with in college—I, however, was profoundly captivated by it. In physics, you won't particularly read anything about God, but you will see the similarities describing *energy* as the same attributes that we have given in describing God. In physics, energy has always existed—it has no beginning or end, it is never trapped by time, it moves freely in and out of dimension, it is in and through every living and non-living thing, and it has the ability to show up in multiple forms at the same time. Doesn't this sound like the characteristics that we also describe as God? In physics, it states that every event has a cause. Isn't the creation of the universe or cosmos considered to be an event—that science calls the Big Bang Theory? Therefore, God or the intelligent mind has to be the *cause* (the energy, Spirit, or life), actuating or putting into action the event. Atheists observing this argument might say that if we believe that every event has a cause, then what made or brought God into existence? And this is a fair question because it is one that I've asked myself most of my life. Let me first admit that every question concerning God cannot be easily explained with observations made only from human or natural perception.

When one asks where did God come from—they do not understand that God is outside of our natural

318

explanations. God or infinite intelligence is not affected by time, space, or matter—because God operates outside of them. Time, space, and matter are what is called in science a "continuum." And these three components must be in existence corresponding at the same time—because if there was the matter—but no space, then **"where"**—would you put the matter? If there was matter and space, but no time—then **"when"** would you put them? You cannot have time, space, and matter existing independently—they must all be present simultaneously in order for creation to happen. And the explanation of there being a God who orchestrates all of this—yet not being affected by any of these factors—is the only thing that makes sense to creation. I reference Genesis 1:1 again. *In the beginning*...represents **"time,"** *God created the heavens...* which represents **"space,"** *and God created the earth*...which represents **"matter."** So, we see that the infinite intelligence that I call God—working in the supernatural realm (outside of our human capacity)—in order to create our natural and physical reality—that we call the world. This is what makes infinite intelligence, God.

If we try and understand God from the observable and empirical frame of reference—we will only run ourselves in circles. In the empirical or logical world, things are measurable and observable—and there are laws in science that support its construct. But the spiritual or supernatural world has its' own laws, too—

though they may not be as clearly understood or discerned from human logic. And we cannot impose the principle of physical laws into the non-physical or supernatural realm—they can never be relevant to one another. Laws applicable to the physical or tangible world cannot be applied to the world of the unseen and intangible. So, we must conclude that the only thing we have close to the explanation in referencing the beginning of all things is what we term God. We must understand or come to believe that God does not need or require a *cause*—in order to be the actuation of effect.

A God of Vengeance & Punishment?

The five major religions of the world are Christianity, Islam, Judaism, Hinduism, and Buddhism—but only Christianity and Islam teach that God is a deity of revenge and retribution. In Christianity, the final place of retribution for *unbelievers* (non-followers of Jesus Christ) is hell. In the Quran, it signifies this place of retribution for *evil-doers* as Jahannam. Judaism does believe in a type of hell, but not one that is the result of eternal fire and brimstone. Judaism does not see hell as a place of punishment, as in the conventional sense—but rather a place or condition of being groomed. Jewish mystics in Judaism describe this spiritual place as Gehinnom—which is translated as hell in Christian texts. But Gehinnom is best translated as the Heavenly Washing Machine because that's exactly how it works. The way a *soul* is cleansed in Gehinnom is similar to the way a shirt would be washed in a washing machine. The shirt would undergo a lot of shaking, agitation, and spinning in hot water, which could be seen as a rough and vigorous process. But the fact is…it is only going through a process so that the shirt can be worn again. Therefore, in Judaism, this is an act of restoration and not retribution.

I am personally more in alignment with the belief of the Buddhist and the Hindu when it comes to the matter of God being vengeful or "retributional." The Buddhist believes that revenge is giving in to anger and self-cherishing and is incompatible with practicing compassion. I cannot imagine a supremely intelligent entity becoming angry or exhausted with its subordinate creation (like human beings) so much as to place them into the ever-lasting fire as a punishment. If we are indeed the creation of what we call God— then how is it that an "all-knowing," omnipotent, intelligent, and compassionate creator would reek that kind of judgment upon its own creation? If the Creator is in all, and through all—just as *energy* is—how could it not know what our actions and outcome will be?

I also ascribe to the beliefs of the Hindu as it relates to God as "not" being an entity of retribution. The Hindu believes in karma and reincarnation and does not recognize the concept of heaven or hell. Nor do they believe in the concept of Satan or the devil because that is in eternal opposition to God as being

"All In All." I agree with the Hindu concept because I personally believe that if God., as physics describes as *eternal energy*—is living and moving in every living thing—how could anything opposing the nature of God be present at the same time? And if it is indeed possible for two opposites to abide in one *being*—then God is both good and evil. Could good and evil simply be constructs orchestrated in our logical realm of explanation for the things we want or don't want in our lives? In other words, are the terms good & evil laws that are only operative in our world of logic and not factors in the world of the spiritual or supernatural? The Hindus believe that all living beings carry a part of Brahman (God) within them. The divine spark/ *energy* is known as atman or soul, and it is immortal. I, too, believe, as I have stated repeatedly throughout this book, that God is as much a part of us as salt is to the sea. There is absolutely no separation of us from the divinity that is within us that we call God. King David stated in Psalm 139:7-10 (paraphrased) *Where can I go that your Spirit won't be present? How can I separate from your presence? If I go into the heavens, you will be there; If I landed in hell or the grave, you would be there too...* And Romans 8:38-39 reads; *For I am persuaded, that neither death, nor life, nor angels, nor principalities, nor powers, nor things present, nor things to come, nor height, nor depth, nor any other creature, shall be able to separate us from the love of God...* So even from the biblical text, we can see that God has no place away from *Its* creation!

What Would Be the Premises for Punishment?

My logical dilemma with the concept of an eternal punishment called hell is its premise? What is the purpose of God in creating a place of eternal retribution? I remember from theology school, the professor addressed this as God giving mankind a choice to be a *free moral agent*. A *free moral agent* or "free will being" is someone who understands the difference between right and wrong and, therefore, can be held responsible for their actions. Even in my twenty-year-old mindset, that whole concept sounded twisted to me. Looking at this concept from a natural manner—and for the sake of making my point— viewing God as a parent—what natural parent would give their five-year-old the choice of a piece of candy or a live grenade? If the Creator of the universe is indeed ALL GOOD as many have ascribed, then why would good and evil be a choice? Why wouldn't everything presented to us be only good? Why, if a person chose evil—would they be subjected to eternal damnation—why would that option even be on the table? Why would punishment even be an aspect of our reality? I thought of the scripture in Mathew 7:9-11 that reads:

What man among you, whose son asked for a piece of bread, would give his son a rock instead? Or if the

323

son asked for a fish, be given a snake instead? If you, as the human parent (sinful in nature), know how to give good and advantageous gifts, how much more will God, who is in heaven and who is perfect, give good gifts to those who ask?

As a parent, if I didn't want my child to have something that would be harmful to them—I would never expose him or her to it. And as a parent, I would not bring a child into the world only to tell them, if you don't do what I want you to do in life—then I will disown you and cast you into a place of punishment. How cruel would that be of me as a parent! So why would a creator expose their creation to something that is considered to be bad or detrimental to them? And what pleasure will the Creator get if its creation chooses the live grenade (given in the earlier example) over the piece of candy and destroys him or herself? I know this might sound like a foolish example, but I believe it makes a strong point. Why would our Creator taunt us with the decisions of pleasure over confinement—understanding that we are free-spirited beings with pleasure-seeking characteristics? Where are we placing our critical thinking skills in these scenarios?

I propose that all holy text is comprised of what I call the "morality factor." Every civilization known to man has established some form of code of conduct for its society in hopes of maintaining a level of proper behavior among its citizens. And there is absolutely nothing wrong with that because a code of conduct in our society is what causes us to be civil towards one another. It is a kind of bridge to maintain harmony. But I believe that too many rules and regulations have been added to civilizations to control or dominate the activities of their societies—all in the name of God! An example of this is that many slave owners demanded that their non-indentured slaves would become Christians because slave owners knew that a slave professing Christianity would be more submissive. It was taught by so-called Christian slave owners that it was the will of God for slaves to obey their masters in all things. This imposed slave code of conduct that was expected and even demanded by slave owners did not allow a slave husband to have any say or opinion when "he" (the master) wanted to sleep with the enslaved husband's wife.

A slave had no choice or voice in a matter if the owner decided to split up the enslaved family—and sell the children. And this, too, was done in the name of God! There are many examples of this kind of religious domination in every culture—but I won't go into them all for the sake of staying on point. Again, the point that I am making is that many laws, rules, regulations, creeds, and proclamations are falsely made in the name of God, the Creator of the universe. And if human beings are indeed *free moral agents*, as my theology professor claimed—then why would the Creator design a concept that doesn't really allow us to be free? The mere fact of *having* to choose between one and another already denounces *free moral agency* or free will—because there is only one good decision to make if one is not willing to "suffer" the consequences of making the wrong choice. Who in their right mind would accept or choose a piece of chocolate cake that they knew was laced with cyanide? No one in their right mind would choose a slice of cake that was laced with poison. Why would the Creator present you with something pleasurable and then tell you that you will go to hell if you partake of it? Why even show you the cake if you can't eat it? So where is the "free will" in this situation for anyone who thinks logically?

I conclude that God is not *necessarily* a deity that is morally-based, but is a God of structure. I personally do not believe that God is concerned over all the little right and wrong deeds that we commit as human beings—the same way a parent does not stress over all the mishaps that their child is going to experience in life. As a parent, we give our children guidelines to live by so that they will become a good person who initiates no harm to others, a good citizen who is law abiding—and someday, maybe a good parent themselves. But we do not keep a record of every wrong they do in their lives so that one day we can rain judgement on them at the end of their lives. As a parent, the purpose of instilling values into our children is not to hinder their enjoyment of life, but to give them a baseline for surviving in a society that recognizes and judge appropriate and inappropriate behavior. In other words, we teach our children *how not to rock the boat* of society norms. And the lessons of survival that we teach our children in America—would not be the same as it would be if we lived in countries like Afghanistan, Yemen, Syria, or Somalia. People's values define what they want personally, but morals define what the society demands from you.

I do believe that God (whom I identify as the Source of all things), is the power or energy that actuates or puts into action everything in and out of our reality. I believe that the Creator God is the power source that fuels every human expectation and drive. God is to humanity what an engine is to a car—for without an engine, a car is only in existence but without functionality. And like a car—our experiences should take us to many places in our current existence. I believe that our life is to be full of experiences—good and bad because these experiences are only a small part of the multiple realities that we will experience in other dimensions. Our lives and experiences are our own—and should not be governed by someone else—as long as we bring no harm to another. Our lives should never *initiate* danger, infringement, or criminality upon others.

The life we desire as human beings are held in the realm of our understanding of how much of God's infused energy within us is utilized. This is to say that an aspect of the Creator resides in each one of us. Therefore, it is up to us as individuals to create and accomplish the life we seek. *For it is God working in you, giving you the desire, power, and "how-to" in pleasing him* (Philippians 2:13). Our Creator understands the purpose of each and every one of us— for we are God's handiwork. However, it may sometimes be unbeknown to us (the creation) what our purpose is. But rest assured that if we allow ourselves to tune into the energy or voice of God within our human vessel—we will hear clear instructions for the path we are to take in this life. I believe we need not judge ourselves from a moral standpoint because we are here on this earth to express God in all of *Its* many facets.

These facets will be viewed as good or bad by the spectators in life—but do not allow the perceptions of others to guide your life. Live your life unto yourself and to the Spirit—with honor and respect for your fellow man. You will make your path prosperous, and you will encounter success in all of your journeys. The Spirit of God will lead you into healthy habits and activities, and you will always find your way back to the waters of peace when you encounter trouble. Listen always to the still, calm voice deep within your being—and you will become like the voice within your soul. In other words, you will become like the God that resides within you. Finally, remember—we can never be separated from God, and God cannot be separated from us. And as I have said before, *God is as much a part of us—as salt is to the sea.* ___

INDEX

Made in the USA
Columbia, SC
02 November 2024

45271109R00183